Mark Rothman's
Essays

ISBN: 978-0-615-43781-1

First Edition: Copyright, February, 2011

Contents

4

Why I Felt The Need To Yell The "F" Word At The Top Of My Voice At A Funeral Home.

Welcome to my essays, which have been culled from my blog over the last two years. My blog can be found at: markrothmansblog.blogspot.com.
The essays found here are for the most part no longer on the blog. This book is pretty much the only way you can find them. But if you like these, there are still plenty to be found that are still at the website.

I have had an interesting life.
Maybe not fascinating.
Maybe I'm not a fascinating person.
Some writers I know think they are so fascinating that they have written four or more autobiographical novels or plays about their own one self.
You always draw from your own life when you write fiction of any kind, but I think it's immodest to make your life the centerpiece of your work.
I have tried to draw on fascinating things that I just happened to experience. Or imagine.
And my goal is simply to tell a ripping yarn as interestingly as possible.
I'm not here to tell you what I had for lunch today.
There are actually blogs that do that.
This is not like twittering.
This is not an ego trip.
I promise that I'll only post something here when I think it will be genuinely of interest to you.

I welcome your responses. My e-mail address is:
macchus999@aol.com

I'm not all that prolific a writer.
I don't get up every day and start writing.
In fact, I almost never write.
Not that I have anything against it.
I've just never been an idea person.
I'm much more an executor.
I get a good idea about once every three years or so.

But when I get one, it's usually totally original, and a
beauty.
And I'm a very fast script-writer.

It usually takes me about three weeks to write a
screenplay or play.
So when you get a good idea once every three years,
and it takes you three weeks to write it, that leaves you
with a lot of free time.
I count on the kindnesses of people who hire me to
write their ideas or do rewrites on existing scripts that
need help.
Except for that, when not on an assignment, I don't
write.

That's primarily why I started writing essays on a
blog.

Now, I'm not proud of yelling "Fuck" at a Funeral
Home.
Nor am I ashamed of it, as my lovely wife would like
me to be. In my mind, circumstances warranted it.

In the winter of 2009, I attended a wake at a Funeral Home.

The deceased was a cousin of mine who died way too young, was a wonderful person, and I was in no way put out by having to attend, even knowing that it was going on the same time as the NFC Championship Game. (I am a huge sports fan.)
Fortunately, there is the wonderful invention called Tivo.

Now, Tivo is no guarantee that I'm going to avoid hearing the score of the game in a public situation. But I figured that a Funeral Home is one of the least likely places to hear it.

There would be people wandering in long after I got there, and they might mouthe off, but I tried to isolate myself, monopolizing the time of people who had arrived when I did.
I thought I had a good shot at pulling it off:

Getting out of there, into my car, and home to watch the game on Tivo.

We stayed for about four hours.
We were about to leave.
My wife said we were going to leave now.
I got my overcoat from the checkroom.
I was five feet from the front entrance-----------my two nieces and two nephews (all in their 20's) enter from outside.
One of the nephews immediately says to me "Uncle Mark, did you root for the Cardinals?"

Now, as any sports fan or anyone who has tried to Tivo a game would know, my nephew's words immediately told me that A- The Cardinals won the game, and B- If you bet on the Eagles, laying the points, as I did, you lost your bet.
A double whammy. I immediately yelled at my nephew " I'm Tivoing the game! Not another word! My God! I was practically out the door!"

My wife, coming to his defense, said "He didn't tell you anything".
"He told me enough!" I snarled.
Then I said the Magic Word.

My nephew knows me well enough to know that I cared about the game, or he wouldn't have said what he said.
And he knew I couldn't have possibly seen the game if I was on my way out the door of a funeral home.
And he's heard of Tivo and knows that I have it.
And he's capable of putting two and two together, and realizing that I might just possibly be Tivoing the game. He wasn't being a wise-ass.
He's a really sweet kid.
And he meant well.
But.....I was practically out the door!!

In the words of just about every 1950's comic, "These kids today!"

Ladies and gentlemen of the jury, I ask you, what would you have done?

*****

My Curse.

In my first essay, I mentioned that, as a writer, I am not an idea person.

I attribute this to a single fact: I have seen just about every movie or TV show worth seeing, and I have an encyclopedic, photographic memory of everything I have seen on the screen.
This is what I consider to be My Curse.

It's very stifling to the imagination when, if you think you have a good idea for a piece of fiction, your mind immediately goes to where that idea was originally done and therefore gets rejected for that reason.

About twenty years ago, a very shrewd screenwriter convinced a major studio to do a comedy about a young married couple and their baby.
The hook was, you could hear the baby's thoughts.
You might remember it. It was called "Look Who's Talking", the baby's thoughts were voiced by Bruce Willis, it was an enormous hit, and spawned a sequel.

If this idea had occurred to me, my first thought would have been "No. I can't pitch that. It's been done. It was a TV sitcom that lasted a season on NBC in 1960 called "Happy". When I was twelve.
And "Happy" was basically a ripoff of an earlier NBC sitcom, "The People's Choice", which starred Jackie Cooper. In it, Jackie had a dog. A basset hound.
And you got to hear the dog's thoughts.
So that would have been the end of it, as far as I was concerned.

The way my mind works, I would have assumed that EVERYBODY remembered "Happy".
But nobody does.
Look at the fortune THAT one cost me.

My Curse.

Also, as a show runner on many sitcoms, I've had all sorts of stories pitched to me.
When I was head writer on the Odd Couple TV series, (No, I'm not a hundred. I was very young when I started.) a writer came in and started pitching a story for Oscar and Felix.
I stopped him after only a few sentences and said "They did this story on the Dick Van Dyke Show".
Sheepishly, he said "Yeah. I know. I wrote it."

My Curse.

But sometimes My Curse leads me to something absolutely fascinating and mind-blowing.

I mentioned in my first essay that fascinating things have happened to me.
When I saw the movie "Revolutionary Road", something really weird happened.

In the 1980's, there was a really interesting series that lasted on NBC for a couple of years called "Crime Story".
It starred Dennis Farina, and was about the Cops vs. the Mob in Chicago and Las Vegas in the late 1950's and early 60's.
There was a recurring character.

I don't even remember whether he was a cop or a mobster.
But the actor made a vivid impression on me.
He just had one of those faces.
I never knew his name, and hadn't seen or thought of him since.

So I'm watching "Revolutionary Road", and there is an actor playing Leonardo DiCaprio's brother-in-law.

I'm looking at him, and he looks remarkably like the above-mentioned actor from "Crime Story".

But this is twenty years later, and the brother-in-law was a contemporary of DiCaprio's.
So it couldn't be him. But boy, does he look like him.
I thought of stopping the DVD and mentioning this to my wife, but I was pretty sure that she never saw "Crime Story", and would think me a lunatic for even bringing it up.
And she would be right.
So I just kept my thoughts to myself, and continued watching.

Literally within the next fifteen minutes, playing another character, the guy who tries to hire away DiCaprio from his current job, the actor from "Crime Story" appeared on the screen.
Looking twenty years older. As he should.
I checked the end credits and noted the actor's name: Jay Sanders.

I immediately went to the Internet, God bless it, and looked him up on the IMDB. The movie database.
There it was: "Crime Story" 1986. Ten Episodes.
I wasn't dreaming. What are the odds?

I looked up the actor who played the brother-in-law.
There seemed to be no relation.

It's not like he said to the director "Hey, you know
who'd be great for this part? My father!"

Pure cosmic coincidence, caused by My Curse.
I will relate other examples of this that have happened
to me over the years.
Too often to chalk up to random happenstance.

This is why I believe there is order in the universe.

*****

When Las Vegas Was Worth It.

The title of this article would imply that Las Vegas is now NOT worth it.
This is an accurate implication.

Las Vegas is now 14 versions of Cirque du Soleil.

Las Vegas is now people lined up around the block 3 times deep to spend way too much to see Celine Deon.

It's Strip traffic that never moves.

It's Siegfried without Roy.

It's a place where someone named Danny Gans was famous.

It's so overbuilt and bloated and mean-spirited that it would be better off if it was robbed of all its personality (which would be petty theft) .

With all the other places in the country to gamble, I really can't fathom why anybody goes there.
It wasn't always that way.

Now, I'm not talking about the Rat Pack Days.
I'm not that old to remember it, although I'm sure it was everything they say it was.

I started going there in the early '70's, and I loved everything about it.
The gambling, the shows, the generosity of the freebies if you gambled, the clean air, the room to breathe....it was really something.
For me, it was what Disneyland is for kids.

And I got to see all the great shows.
And all the cheezy shows.
For free.

And even the cheezy shows had something wonderfully awful about them.

There were two performers of whom it was always said "I know they don't seem like much on TV, but you have to see them live"----Wayne Newton and Shecky Greene.

Well, I got to see them both live in Vegas in the '70's. And they were both perfectly awful.

Wayne Newton wasn't any less schlocky, and Shecky Greene worked so hard for the four laughs he got over the course of an hour-and-a-half that I really felt bad for him.

But I wouldn't have missed either of them for the world.

Capsule reminiscences:

Elvis. Great. Mostly, you were overwhelmed by the event.

Streisand. Ditto.

Rodney. Always pissing funny. Saw him probably four times. Always different material.

Cosby. Did less than an hour, seated in an easy chair. With no opening act.
Completely phoned it in. Probably just an off-night.

Sammy. I don't know, I just didn't get it.
I've seen him in other contexts, where he was magnificent.
"Golden Boy" on Broadway in the '60's.
Sensational.
He made some great recordings.
He was a wonderful actor.
He certainly was amazingly talented and versatile.

But in this venue, it just didn't work for me.
I was seated in a booth with 3 women I didn't know,
and they were just gushing throughout.
I kept thinking "What?!"
I just couldn't get past the phoniness.
I guess I just turned out not to be a fan of Sammy
Davis in Concert.
Not his fault.
All these things are subjective.
I went mainly to see Rosemary Clooney, who opened
for him.
She was magnificent.

Tony Bennett. Less is more.
He did over two hours, and it felt repetitious after an
hour.
Rosemary Clooney used to mock-complain that
whenever she was up for a Grammy, she'd lose to
Tony Bennett.
But the Grammy voters were right.
Tony Bennett was a much better recording artist, and
Rosemary Clooney was far superior in person.

Bob Newhart. Completely professional, polished,
genuinely funny, delightful.

Alan King. Ditto.

George Carlin. Always funny, but the material
invariably showed up on his next HBO special. He
used Vegas to break it in.
And he always had a bad opening act.

Liza. If you sit too close, you could see the sweat
pouring off of her.

If you saw her more than once in the run, you were
aware that she does precisely the same show every
night.

Spontaneity does not exist.

Rickles. Saw him three times. Invariably disappointing.
I think I kept going back because I figured "It has to be me".
You don't want to sit close enough to the stage to become a target.

Rickles was funny when he was Nobody picking on Somebody.
Or Nobody picking on Nobody.
Or Somebody picking on Somebody.
When he was on Carson or Dean Martin, he was great.
When he's on Letterman or Leno, he's great.
I'm sure when he was a Lounge comic picking on drunks, he was great.
But when I saw him in Vegas, he was this Big Star picking on tourists.

It's overkill, and embarrassing.
The Emmy-winning documentary about him captured it pretty accurately, but there's no reason for him to be proud of it.

Sinatra. Magic. Awesome.
Saw him three times. Always sensational.
One of those times, Count Basie and Ella Fitzgerald appeared with him.
Permit me a digression: Am I the only one in the United States who doesn't see what the shouting is about with Ella Fitzgerald?
Yes, she's a quite technically proficient scat-singer.
But no better than Mel Torme.
Her attempts at ballads are always sugary, syrupy, and completely devoid of personality.
I've never known anything about this woman through her music, other than her reputation as Madame Queen.

Why other singers and musicians roll over and play
dead for her is beyond me.
What am I missing?
Louis Prima. We will never see his likes again, and
that's a damned shame.

Harry Belafonte. Ditto.

Buddy Hackett. Easily the most consistently,
explosively funny Vegas comedian ever.
Saw him like four times.
One time stands out, for a couple of reasons.
Danny Thomas showed up to watch him, with what
appeared to be a thousand-a-night hooker on his arm.
I was with a couple of my less-than-hip friends who
couldn't believe what they were seeing.
Mr. Wholesome. Mr. Family Man. Mr. Make Room
For Daddy.
I said "Believe it".
One of the friends, clutching at perhaps one too many
straws, said, out loud, I swear, "Maybe she's a friend
of Marlo's".
I swear.

The other reason it stands out is that three days later I
was back in L.A., hanging out at the Comedy Store.
This was in its early days. When it was a breeding
ground for Letterman, Robin Williams, really great
people.
I saw Richard Pryor there once.

A comedian was announced, got up on stage, and
immediately launched into Buddy Hackett's act,
verbatim.
The same material I just saw three days previously.
And he was bombing with it.
That only slightly mitigated my outrage.
I felt like standing up and shouting "You're doing
Buddy Hackett's act! Badly!"

I restrained myself.

But I made sure to catch his name after he got done.

The emcee said "How about a nice hand for Kenny Kramer, folks".

I decided to remember that name and that face.
I was already in a position to decide who to cast or not cast on the sitcoms I was working on, and he was never to get in the door.

Cut to: The '90's. Seinfeld's show became popular.
Entertainment Tonight sought out the real Kramer.
The one the character was based on.
Or, more likely, he sought them out.
They interviewed him.
Hopefully you are ahead of me at this point.
Yes, it was Kenny Kramer.

He was trying to cash in on Seinfeld's success by conducting guided tours of Seinfeld haunts.

It was very nice to see him not doing too well.

*****

The Nude Beach.

I consider myself to be an expert on Nude Beach Behavior.

I spent the better part of the '90's living at Lake Tahoe, spending the better part of ten years at its nude beach.
It's actually a clothing optional beach, which can present some problems.

There is usually some unspoken resentment by the nudists towards the people who wear at least a bathing suit.
Being the conformist that I am, I usually went with the daily majority.

If there were more naked people than not, my pants would come off.
If they were outnumbered, I'd keep them on.

Through experience, I have learned that there are two reasons, or a combination of two reasons, why people go to the nude beach.
It has nothing to do with not wanting a tan line, or to be totally at one with nature.

It's to see or be seen by members of the sex that interested them, naked.

In my case, it has been to see as many women in that state, starting out dressed, and ending up undressed.

I have found nudists to be a generally weird lot. Many are very uptight at being stared at, which begs the question "Then why are you dropping your drawers in public?"
The question "What are you lookin' at?" is one I've heard far more often than you might think.

It's really not sexual.
I've never experienced an erection there, nor have I ever seen any male experience one.

Perhaps it's the elephant in the room (or the lake), but it has never been an issue.

I once witnessed a young couple having an enormous heated verbal exchange, ending in them not talking to each other.
Naked.
I found this dynamic hilarious.

I once saw The Amazing Kreskin, the "mentalist", at the nude beach.
I didn't know him, but that didn't stop me from going up to him and saying "Hello Kreskin".
He, in full Kreskin voice, refused to admit that he was, indeed, Kreskin.
Indeed he was.
But, for the record, he wasn't all that Amazing, if you get my drift.

I've written an entire screenplay, and an entire play at the nude beach.
It's a very good test for you as a writer.
If you can concentrate on the page, with all the pulchritude around you, you must really be on a roll, and really be on to something.

Being somewhat averse to sand, I would usually pump up a life raft, take it out on the water, armed with my yellow legal pad and a pen, and write.

One day, I was out on my raft, writing away, and I noticed a young couple in their 20's descending the huge incline leading to the floor of the nude beach.
The girl was absolutely gorgeous.
They planted themselves directly in front of where I had left my bag of stuff.

They begin disrobing.
The girl had a phenomenal body.
She sits down, completely naked, and removes from her beach bag an enormous black bonnet, with a huge brim, and bows enabling her to tie the bonnet around her neck.
She puts it on her head, and ties the bow.
From the neck up, she looked like a Renoir portrait.
In a master shot, she looked ridiculous.

So I'm sitting out there on the raft, and I'm thinking "I've got the line.
All I need is the opportunity to use it".

At around 3pm, the Lake started getting choppy.
This was a common occurrence around this time of day.
This made it impossible to keep writing.
So I paddle my way to shore, and plant myself directly behind girl with the bonnet.
And I'm waiting for the opportunity.
And I'm waiting.
And I'm waiting.

Finally, she starts to untie the bow and remove the bonnet.
The opportunity was at hand.

I said, out loud, "Don't take off the hat! It makes the whole outfit!"

The fifteen or so people within earshot laughed hysterically.

Never will I be better set up for a one-liner.

*****

How Do You Break Into The Business?

This is the question I'm asked most frequently and usually first whenever I do a lecture, or begin teaching a writing or acting class, both of which I do on occasion.
I am one of the least qualified people to answer that question.
This is because the circumstances of my Breaking In were quite uncommon, to say the least.

I grew up in New York City. The Bronx, then Queens, to be specific.
When I was in the sixth grade, there was this thing called the "S.P.'s"---special progress classes.
There was this test you had to take to determine whether or not you'd make the "S.P.'s."
If you made the "S.P.'s", you'd skip the 8th grade.
You'd go right from the 7th to the 9th.
Every kid's mother put a ton of pressure on every kid to study hard to make the "S.P.'s"
If you didn't, you'd bring shame to the family. Or "A shanda fa duh Schrayna", as my mother so eloquently put it in Yiddish, rolling her R's on "Schrayna".
As Reader's Digest would put it, "Towards More Picturesque Speech".
Knowing she would slit her wrists, or stick her head in the oven, I strove mightily to make the "S.P.'s".
We all took the test, and waited in dread for the results.
There were 5 classes in the 6th grade in my school, and I was in the second smartest.
You knew this because the Public School system made no bones about telling you.
Damn nice of them.
And there was no subtlety about it.

The classes were 6-1, 6-2, 6-3, 6-4, and 6-5. I was in
6-2.

Everybody knew the score.

Except maybe the kids in 6-5.

One afternoon, a couple of weeks later, the Assistant
Principal, Miss Steiner, a harridan if you ever saw one,
came into our classroom with a bunch of index cards
in her hands.

You wanna hear about a sadist?

She announced " The following children have made
the "S.P.'s".

She started reading alphabetically.

We were seated alphabetically.

The entire first row made it.

The first 3 in the second row made it.

The next name was skipped.

The kid was crushed.

The next 4 made it.

The next name was skipped.

That kid was crushed.

It pretty much held that pattern.

They got to the R's.

They got to me.

My name was skipped.

The word "suicide" entered my brain for the first time.

The harridan got to the alphabetical end.

Then she started calling off names, still reading from
the index cards.

Names she had skipped alphabetically.

She read my name.

My thoughts of razor blades and gas jets disappeared.

The shrew then went on and on, until she had named
every last member of our class.

We all made the "S.P's".

Now, what motivates a person to do things this way,
besides outright cruelty?!

She should have been brought up on charges.

So I made the "S.P.'s" I went home and told my
mother, who immediately launched into three
choruses of "Zip-A-Dee-Doo-Dah".

It turned out to be the worst thing that ever happened.
To those who didn't make it, for psychological
reasons, and those who did, like me, for practical
ones.
If you made the S.P.'s, you were a virtual lock for
college, and this meant you started college at 16.
Who's ready for college at 16?
What college co-ed is going to want to go out with a 16
year-old?
But off I went, to Queens College.
A very good school. And as one of the City colleges, it
was virtually a free education.
But the kids who didn't make the "S.P's" really got the
best of it.
They were ready for college when they got there, they
had social lives, and their grades were better.
Better than mine, anyway.
I nearly flunked out at the end of the first year.

Then something miraculous happened.
I met a fellow student who told me there was a
Theatre Department on campus.
I, as a walking fetus, did not know that.
I love the theatre (and never come late).
I auditioned for plays, and got cast.
There were girls in these plays.
Girls who would talk to you.
The next semester, I signed up for theatre classes.
More girls.
I started getting A's.
More A's. More plays. More girls.
Girls who wouldn't give me the time of day, whom I
could cop a feel off of because it said so in the script.

I worked my average all the way up to a C at one point.
It took me six years, but I finally got my B.A. in theatre, which, as we all know, is a Passport to Nowhere.

What does this have to do with breaking into show business?

 Okay. If you start college at 16, and spend 6 years there, with a theatre degree, no money, and no steady job, that makes you 22, and still living at home.
That was me.

In the last two years of my college stay, I was encouraged by some of my friends to join their House Plan.
A House Plan is basically a Fraternity without the hazing and beer.

They were usually a little nerdier than Frats, and ours was easily the nerdiest on campus.
But we were more democratic than most.
We would accept anybody.
And I mean An-Nee-Bod-Dee.

You should have seen some of the pathetic creatures we provided a home for.

Our House Plan was important to us for three main reasons:

1) Poker.

2) Futilely trying to meet girls,
and

3) An annual event that was held called "Frolics".Frolics was a competition held among about 7 or 8 male House Plans.

Each was teamed up with a female House Plan.
Each pair would put on a 15 minute original mini-
musical.
There would be first-prize, second-prize, and third
prize trophies.

It was held in the campus's huge 2000-seat
auditorium, which was always filled to the brim for
this event.

This was a Large Deal.

Now, I had attended Frolics the year before I joined
the House Plan.
I found the sketch that my future House Plan put on
to be quite funny, but I thought that the songs were
dreadful.
So did they.
They finished fifth.
The sketch-writer (NOT the songwriter) and I were
already quite chummy.
I'd known him off and on since I was twelve and he
was eleven.
He was and is one of the funniest people in the world.
Right up there with Mel and Albert Brooks.
He was and is Lowell Ganz.
Maybe you've heard of him.
He was the main reason I joined the House Plan.
Every school day, he'd hold court in the cafeteria, with
all the rest of us nerds, hilariously hurling invectives
in every direction.
Except mine.
Shrewdly, he realized that I wouldn't be all that
receptive.
And I wasn't as easy a target.
But the others lapped it up as a Badge of Honor.
As if they were being insulted by Rickles.
I'm sure it was better than the Algonquin Round
Table.

Now, this was the late 60's, and there were a lot of
great shows running in New York.
Hello Dolly.
Cabaret.
Fiddler On The Roof.

But Lowell in the Queens College cafeteria was easily
the Best Show In Town.

He was the Cyrano De Bergerac of Abuse.

So my joining the House Plan was inevitable.

Frolics was coming around.
Being known as somewhat musical, I was recruited to
write the songs and Lowell would write the dialogue
for the coming year's sketch, which we determined to
be a 12 and a half minute version of "Gone With The
Wind".
I had already built a minor reputation for musical
chops by having written and performed a little ditty
entitled "Horseradish".
In some circles, I am better known and admired for
"Horseradish" than for any of my other work.
After one brief session with him, we both decided that
we would co-write the dialogue.
We complemented each other, made each other
better, and were totally on the same wave-length.
I managed to work "Horseradish" into the sketch.
Organically.
I directed it, and played the banjo. Lowell played
Scarlett's father, and sang "Horseradish".

The President of Frolics (yes, there was such a
person), whose former job was Vice-President In
Charge of Looking Down His Nose At Us, attended
one of our later rehearsals.

He suggested, then pleaded with us, to drop out.
He thought what he saw was God-Awful.

I looked at him, and with all sincerity, said
"No. Sheldon, you don't understand. We're going to
win this thing."
Very Joe Namath-like of me.
And the outcome was the same as Broadway Joe's.

The nerdiest guys, matched up with the nerdiest girls
(who still far outclassed us), with virtually no budget
for sets or costumes (All the guys wore their Bar-
Mitzvah suits with the lapels turned up. There were
still yarmulkes in the pockets. And we were doing the
Civil War.) won First Prize.
It was pandemonium. Still the highlight of many
people's lives.
Somewhere, out there, Sheldon is probably still
whimpering.

We came back and did it again the next year, only this
time the snootier girl groups were clamoring to be
matched up with us.

At this point, Lowell and I, continually trying to deal
with the question "What kind of work are we out of?"
decided we were out-of-work writers.

Almost every weekday evening, he and I would
congregate at Lowell's parents' apartment, where, of
course, he still lived, early enough for Mrs. Ganz to
offer me dinner, which I would gratefully accept.
My mother worked, and had long been out of the
business of making me dinner.
The word "nuchshlepper" was already starting to be
thrown around liberally at my house by my mother,
and directed toward me.

(For the uninformed, "nuchshlepper" is Yiddish for
one who takes advantage of another by riding
another's coattails.)

Yiddish is a pretty colorful language.

At 6:30, Channel 9 would have reruns of the Dick Van Dyke Show.
We loved it, and watched it religiously.
Every night, at 6:45, Lowell's father would trudge up the stairs, after a hard day's work, and a commute that required him to take the subway and two buses.
He'd look at us as we were watching Van Dyke and say, like clockwork, "You're gonna make a living from this?"

Little did he know.

Then God fell into our laps.
In the form of my father, who, to his credit, never called me a nuchshlepper.

After being a cab-driver for much of his adult life, he decided to go into the Limousine business.
The occasional work that I did do was usually driving a limousine for my father's business, which made very little sense, since I was and am probably the worst driver who was ever issued a license.
Second only to my mother, who WAS the worst.
Apples and trees.
Once, in Columbus Circle in midtown Manhattan, right near Dick Cavett's TV studio, on the way to the Cavett show with Dr. Martin Luther King's second in command, Rev. Ralph Abernathy in the back seat, I drove into oncoming traffic.
The oncoming drivers mercifully all put on their brakes, and the Civil Rights Movement wasn't stifled any further.
I have never been in an accident.
But God knows how many I must have caused.

My father was a very charming man.
He had the gift of making people like him.

Primarily because of his charm, and his yearning to be around Show Business, he managed to snare just about every Limousine account for every TV talk show coming out of New York.
And there were a lot of them in 1971.
Carson was still there. Merv Griffin, Dick Cavett.
Mike Douglas had a show in Philadelphia that required a lot of limo work back and forth from New York.
My father had the limo accounts for ALL of these shows, and did most of the driving.

And he was very encouraging about my writing.
I think he was just happy that I was finally showing an interest in doing ANYTHING.
Also, I think he saw it as a way of getting me out of his house sooner.

One day, he said to me "You know, I think I can help you. I get virtually everybody in Show Business in the limo. And I usually know about a week in advance who's going to be in the car.
Why don't I tell you, and you can write material for them?"

We took it from there.
We wrote monologues for Dick Cavett. My father handed them to him.
Nothing.
He had Carol Burnett in the car. We wrote a sketch.
He handed it to her.
Nothing.
Dean Martin. Another sketch.
Nothing.
It went on like this for a few months, not really a long time.
He mentioned us to Mike Douglas, who actually seemed eager to see if we could write a sketch for him.
He wanted to branch out.

We wrote a take-off of "Butch Cassidy and the Sundance Kid" for Mike Douglas.
And we specifically wrote a part for Henny Youngman.
Don't ask why.
But we thought the sketch was very good.

They did it.

And they completely butchered it.

Welcome to Show Business.

Butch and Sundance were played by Mike and Robert Morse.
I forget who played who.
I'm trying to forget everything about it.
Peggy Cass played the Katherine Ross part.
To this day, I cannot look at Robert Morse or Peggy Cass without getting nauseous.
It was all about forgetting their lines, and how silly it was for them to be doing a sketch.
And they shot it without a live audience, but showed it to the audience during the actual taping. .
Another form of death.

But Henny Youngman was great.
It was all I had to cling to.

We thought it was all over for us.
See, we were so dumb that we thought the entire industry was watching.
And that they'd actually remember our names.
But Mike was pleased.
So much so that he invited us to write more sketches.
And to write material for his upcoming Las Vegas Act.
He was going to play Vegas for the first time.
It was also his last time.
But, again, not our fault.
So Mike Douglas was our first paying gig.

Wasn't a fortune, but it impressed the neighbors and relatives.
Literally weeks after that, within the span of a week, My father had Tony Randall in the car, who was guesting with Cavett.

He also had Jack Klugman, who was co-hosting the Mike Douglas Show.
We knew this a week in advance.
The Odd Couple had just finished its second season, and they were on hiatus before starting a third.
So we wrote an Odd Couple episode.
We had never attempted to write a sitcom episode before, but we had all them Van Dyke's under our belts.
We felt we had to have picked up something, just by osmosis.
We didn't really watch the Odd Couple, because it was on Friday nights, and Friday nights meant we were still down at the House Plan, pathetically trying to meet girls, with the added wrinkle of trying to impress them with our meager writing credits.
But we knew the play and the movie. How different could it be?
So we shlepped into Manhattan, to the Lincoln Center Library, to look at the last two years worth of back copies of TV Guide to see what stories they had done.
It was time consuming.
Remember. We only had a week.
Where was the Internet when we needed it?
But we accomplished our mission, and wrote something we thought Neil Simon might be proud of.
My father does his job.
One copy to Tony. One copy to Jack.

A week later, my sister and I go into Manhattan and see the Saturday Matinee of Phil Silvers in "A Funny Thing Happened On the Way to the Forum".
We come home.

My mother and father are arm-whipping each other into the walls. Repeatedly.

"Jack Klugman called the house!", my mother shrieked.
"He wants you to call him!" she again shrieked.
Then there was more shrieking, in general.
So I call Jack Klugman.
He doesn't want to buy the script.
He wants to hire us as staff writers.
This is better than buying the script.
What had taken place was that Jack and Tony each read the script, each loved it, and each called Garry Marshall with the instructions "Hire these guys!!"
We were being flown, first-class, to L.A., with jobs waiting for us.
My nuchshlepping days were over.

The irony is that until about five years ago, when we were all reminiscing backstage in New York, when I saw them in "The Sunshine Boys", neither one of them knew that the other had called Garry Marshall.
Each one thought that he was solely responsible for my success.

I had just brought it up in passing, and they were both stunned.

So, how do you break into the business?

All I can say is, make the S.P's, nearly flunk out of college, be absolutely no good at anything else, have some talent, and have a father who's a limo driver, who can get your work to everyone in Show Business.

And pray. Sorry, that's the best I can do.

*****

Odd CUPPle!!

Earlier, I mentioned that my job experience before I got my career break was severely limited.

This isn't entirely true.

For a couple of summers, when I was still going to college, I was a page at ABC.
This was interesting, and I'll have more to say about that later.

For a couple of other summers, also while still in college, I acted in Dinner Theater tours in the South.
Places like Nashville, Tampa, Greensboro North Carolina, Marietta Georgia.

It was easy for me to get cast.
The responses I got when I acted in college plays were very encouraging, particularly for comedies, and I found that I had the ability to cold-read a script sight-unseen as well as anyone ever could.
This gave me several legs up for Dinner Theater auditions, where they almost exclusively did comedies.
And they cast them out of New York, so I had easy access.

Three things stand out in my Dinner Theater experiences.
Four, if you count the girls.

First, they made all the cast members stand in a receiving line in the lobby after each performance.
It was 300 people coming up to you individually, shaking your hand, and saying " 'njoyed it."
All in the same monotone.

Second, the food was really good.

And we were all invited to participate in the buffet
before the performance.
And I, of course, was a glutton.
It was like going to a Southern-Fried Bar Mitzvah
every night.
And the management put no restrictions on how
much we could eat.
I learned later on from an actor who followed me in
the very next show to be done at Greensboro that as a
result of the show I put on at the buffet, restrictions
were then imposed on every subsequent cast.

My legacy.

Third was the month I played Tampa, Florida.
These Dinner Theaters were franchised, and shared
something in common:
They were all theater-in-the-round, and each had an
elevated platform that was lowered hydraulically until
it reached ground level, where it became the stage.
Rather innovative, I thought.
It was the equivalent of the curtain going up.

Two other actors and I were seated on this raised
platform before it was lowered at the beginning of the
play, because we were all on stage as the play began.

Because of our audible proximity to what went on
below us, we were subjected to the nightly
embarrassment of listening to the owner of the
theater, an old Jewish guy, with a heavy accent named
Billy Rose (No, not THE Billy Rose) do a warm-up for
the audience.
He had a bad toupee.
He told bad jokes.
He had an organist to entertain the crowd and to
punctuate Billy's birthday and anniversary
announcements with "Happy Birthday To You" and
"The Anniversary Waltz".

And the anniversary couple was coaxed on to the dance floor, which the platform eventually covered.

Billy would invariably end his warmup promoting the next show that was coming to the theater.
"And don't forget, folks. Next month we're gonna have Odd CUPPle......"
Always the accent on the CUPP.
Never using the word "The".
Always "Next month we're gonna have Odd CUPPle....."

Three years later, I was on the writing staff of "The Odd Couple".
I figured I had a good audience for this story.
I did.
From then on, every Friday night, as we headed down to the stage for the filming, one of the writers, sometimes me, would say, "Okay, let's do Odd CUPPle....."
It was ritualistic.

Years later, there was a revival of the series called "The New Odd Couple".
Essentially a black version, starring Ron Glass and Demond Wilson.
I ran that show too.
I regaled that writing staff with the Billy Rose story as well.
From then on, it became "Let's do New Odd CUPPle......"

Several years after that, I ran a show called "She's The Sheriff", starring Suzanne Somers.
I had many of the same writing staff that I had on New Odd CUPPle.

In the pilot episode, we had a big scene where Suzanne's character was going to appear on "Nightline", with Ted Koppel.
We didn't actually use Ted Koppel, but rather one of our writers who did a dead-on vocal impression of him, and we put a red wig on him and shot the back of his head.
He was great, and the show was hilarious.
And on our way down to the stage, one of the writers, who had been with me in previous incarnations, turned and said to me "Okay, let's do Ted KOPPel......"

My evening was made before it had begun.

More on both of these shows later on.

I remember, on one of those nights in Tampa, waiting for Billy Rose to get through with his spiel, saying to the other two actors up there on the platform with me, "You know, it's times like these that I get the feeling that maybe we're not in the same business as the Lunts".

*****

Fine Corinthian Leather.

I never worked with Ricardo Montalban, nor did I
ever meet him.
But I heard stories from a very reliable source.
In this case, the reliable source was the late Bob
Denver.
That's right. Gilligan. Maynard G. Krebs.
THAT Bob Denver.
Bob HAD worked with Ricardo. On a "Fantasy Island,
or a "Love Boat", or a "Murder, She Wrote", or
something.

One thing you should know about Bob.
He was ABSOLUTELY NOTHING like the characters
he played.
He was studious, intelligent, articulate, fun to be
around, worldly, a total gentleman, and a wonderful
actor.
Which is exactly how he described Ricardo
Montalban.

According to Bob, nobody in show business ever had a
bad word to say about Ricardo.
And Ricardo never, ever had a bad word to say to or
about anyone.

Except Herve Villechaise.

For the only time in Ricardo's life, it was oil and
water.
The Cobra and the Mongoose.

Herve called him "Boss" when he said "De plane,
boss!" De Plane!"
So I guess that made him "De Employee".

It will be easier to refer to him that way than as something more disparaging that would be politically incorrect about his size, which I'm sure I'd lapse into otherwise.

Anyway, De Employee would drive the usually charming and unflappable Ricardo absolutely berserk with his unprofessionalism and complaining.
De Employee would always show up late on the set, usually hung over, smoking like a chimney, never knowing his lines.
And he bellyached about anything and everything.

In the Walt Disney cartoons, Goofy would on occasion break into song, with a little tune that began "Oh, the World Owes Me a Living...."
This was De Employee's actual life credo.
Late one afternoon, a few years into the run, De Employee sent the crew into Golden Time because of all his stumbling, unpreparedness, and crabbing.
After years of mounting frustration, Ricardo had had enough.

He picked up De Employee by the lapels of his little white tuxedo, and carried him all the way from the Island set to his dressing room, where he literally threw him against the wall, still holding on to him, and began his one and only verbal tirade:

"Listen to me, you miserable replica of humanity! You gnome!
Don't you have any conception of how lucky you are??!!
Do you have any idea how many little shits there are out there, just like you, with probably at least as much talent, who have to work in the circus? Or in carnivals? While you're making thousands of dollars a week?

You could be out there panhandling!
And should be!

You should be down on your little knees, thanking
God, counting your fucking blessings!
Every day of your fucking little life!

Now get out there, cut the shit, and finish the scene so
we can all go home!!"
With that he dropped him to the ground, drop-kicking
him in the seat of his little white pants, right out of his
dressing room.

From that moment on, De Employee really knew who
was De Boss.

Late in his life, Desi Arnaz used to make frequent
appearances on talk shows.
He would often do this very funny routine where he
would describe the history of his life, in sequence, and
in Spanish, punctuated with key words in English. It
would go something like this: (Bear in mind that my
Spanish isn't too good.)

"Cocheta-cocheta-cocheta-cocheta got outta Cuba on a
boat,
Cocheta-cocheta-cocheta-cocheta formed a band,
Cocheta-cocheta Babaloo!!,
Cocheta-cocheta-cocheta-cocheta on Broadway,
"Too Many Girls", more Babaloo,
Cocheta-cocheta-cocheta RKO,
Cocheta-cocheta met Lucy, ay caramba!!
Cocheta-cocheta-cocheta signed with MGM,
Cocheta-cocheta-cocheta went no place,
Cocheta-cocheta-cocheta Montalban, out out out...., "

It went on from there, but for me it peaked with
"Montalban, out out out....,".

Just a few weeks ago, I'd told my wife the Desi Arnaz story.
It tickled her risibilities.

Last night, we were driving home from her mother's and we had the Sirius radio's Broadway station playing.

Ethel Merman was singing "Some People" from the Original Cast album of "Gypsy".
I mused out loud about how great she must have been in that show, and what a shame it was that she didn't do the movie version.

My wife said "You mean she wasn't even offered it?"
I said "Nope. And supposedly it broke Ethel's heart. The way I understand it is that Rosalind Russell's husband used some skullduggery to wangle away the movie rights for his wife.
The result was definitely not an upgrade".

And from out of nowhere, my wife said "Rosalind Russell, out out out....."

It pays to be married.

*****

Why I'm Glad They Blew Up the Sands Hotel.

Remember the movie "Ocean's Eleven"?
No, not the one with George Clooney and no story to
speak of.
I was in Vegas when they were shooting that movie.
Elliot Gould was in it.
One evening, I was walking outside, around the
entrance to the Belaggio, and Elliot Gould was
walking right towards me.
Now, you've got to understand that ever since I was a
young adult, I have borne a very strong resemblance
to Elliot Gould.
I have actually been mistaken for him on several
occasions.
It used to be ""Hey, aren't you Elliot Gould?".
Now, with the younger generation, it's "Hey, aren't
you the guy who plays Ross's father on 'Friends'?".
So he's walking right towards me. We are face to face.
Except I'm a few inches taller, so he's looking up at
me. So I say "Does anybody ever tell you that you look
like me?" He laughed.

No, I'm talking about the legendary "Ocean's Eleven",
with Frank Sinatra and the Rat Pack, with a pretty
good story, and a lot of cheesy acting and dialogue.
The actor Richard Conte had a significant part in it.
Robert Evans, in his autobiography, "The Kid Stays In
the Picture", described his close friendship with famed
producer Mike Todd.
According to Evans, Mike Todd was a great Gin
Rummy player, and taught Evans how to play.
As good a Gin Rummy player as Mike Todd was, he'd
always lose to his friend Richard Conte, whom he
described as the greatest Gin Rummy player of
all-time.

Todd used to say "He should have only been as good an actor as he was a Gin Rummy player".

The movie also had Dean Martin singing that great rendition of "Ain't That a Kick in the Head".

And Sammy Davis, dressed as a garbageman, singing the totally forgettable (except by me) "Ee-o-ee-leven".

It was about them staging a New Year's Eve heist at the five main Las Vegas Strip Hotels at the time:
The Sands
The Desert Inn
The Sahara
The Flamingo
and the Riviera.

These hotels all had one thing in common, beside their status.
They were all very classy places, considering it was Vegas.

There was almost a quiet, staid elegance about them, that's reflected in the movie.
They had dark, wood-paneled walls, soft lighting, and dealers who were outfitted with a distinct dignity.

Even in the 70's, when I started going to Vegas, whenever I went to any of those hotels, I felt underdressed.
I should go up to the room, and put on nicer clothes.

With Vegas becoming the humongous monster it has become, what has happened to those five hotels from Ocean's Eleven?

Well, the first two got blowed up.   As they used to say on that SCTV sketch with John Candy and Joe Flaherty, "They got blowed up real good!".

The other three surviving hotels all went the same route:
The wood-paneled walls were replaced by wall-to-wall neon, the lighting became harsh, the slot machines make WAY too much noise, the blackjack dealers' outfits are garish, most of the women blackjack dealers wear way too much makeup, have two-toned hair, and have WAY too many tattoos.

It was clear that they were now aiming for the RV crowd.

You couldn't possibly feel underdressed any more.
Even if you were in your underwear.

If you walk or drive past the Riviera these days, you are struck by the logos plastered on the front of the building, where just behind lurks the Food Court.
Logos for McDonald's. Burger King, KFC, etc.
Not how I want to remember the Riviera.

The Sahara, former home of Louis Prima and Rickles in the Lounge, and Buddy Hackett and Johnny Carson in the Main Room (and Mike Douglas that one time,-- see "How Do You Break Into the Business? "-- now just looks astoundingly cheap and seedy.

The Flamingo survived less disastrously.
Just much bigger and glitzier.

The Desert Inn at least had the decency to die with some of it's dignity intact.

But the saddest case of all was the Sands.

Not only was it THE classiest, but before it got blowed up real good, it became THE cheesiest.
THE gaudiest.
THE loudest.
THE cheapest.

The rooms were dilapidated. I couldn't imagine Frank even wiping his feet in the nicest suite they had. The biggest Fall from Grace you could possibly imagine.

In the waning days of the Sands, an act played in its open-curtained, slot-machine-distracting, people-continuously-walking-right-past-it Lounge.

A great act.

I hope you remember them.

They were The Limeliters.
Usually billed, somewhat facetiously, but deservingly, as the Fabulous Limeliters.

One of the great Folksinging groups from the Hootenanny Era.

And they had a great sense of humor that was sorely lacking in most other Folk Acts.
Two of the three original members were still there, including the now late Lou Gottlieb, who, if you remember them, was the tall, bespectacled, extremely funny one.
The one who did all the talking.

Two drink Minimum.
I went in, and returned for all three sets.

They were great.
But I felt so badly for them.
You could tell that they were clearly put off by their surroundings, and collectively would have preferred to be anywhere else.

After the last set, they started packing up their instruments, and I headed to the casino.

A few minutes later, I spotted Lou Gottlieb walking
with his covered bass fiddle through the casino.
I stopped him, to speak to him.
I said "I just sat through three sets."
He said "I know."
Due to my size, the sparseness of attendance, and
length of my stay, I wasn't too hard to spot.
"You guys are still great." I said.
He thanked me.
I continued, "But how could you stand it? I mean,
you're the Limeliters, for God's sake.
You shouldn't have to do gigs like this."
He bowed his head, sadly, and said, stoically,
"Sometimes, one must do what one must do."
I felt sorry that I had intruded.

This all begs the question, "If it was so awful at the
Sands, why did you keep going there?"
Let's just say "I had my reasons", and leave it at that.

I have one other vivid memory of the Sands.
This was back in its wood-paneled heyday.
It was the 80's.

I was having dinner in the Sands great Gourmet
restaurant, the aptly named Oak Room.
For free, of course.
I was a high enough roller to warrant that.
Being freshly divorced, I was alone.
Close by, at the head of a long table, the well-known
sportscaster Al Michaels was holding court, with his
family filling the other seats.
It was his birthday, and one by one, each family
member paid glowing tribute to him, and then he paid
glowing tribute to each of them.
It was all very glowing.

As MY family had just been savagely broken up, the
whole thing made me nauseous.

And I tore into my very-well-prepared steak with a vengeance.
But I was genuinely happy for him.

Al Michaels is NOW "the well-known sportscaster".
When he was at the Oak Room, he wasn't all THAT well-known.
He'd already made his bones with "Do you believe in miracles?" when covering the stunning upset of the Russian hockey team by the U.S. team in the 1980 Winter Olympics.
But besides that, I mostly knew him as the voice of the San Francisco Giants.
I had a house in Carmel, California, and we picked up the Giant games all the time.
I do and did think he's a GREAT sportscaster.
When I saw him that night in the Oak Room, his most high profile gig was as the host and play-by-play man for the Back-Up game for ABC's Monday Night Baseball.

The Back-Up game was the game you saw if the Main game was rained out.
Or if you lived in one of the two cities that the two teams playing in the Main Game were from.

Howard Cosell hosted the Main Game.
Al Michaels hosted the Back-Up game.
Definitely less prestigious.

Later on that night, I was in the casino.
I saw Al Michaels at one of the Crap Tables, betting red five-dollar chips.

I don't play Craps. I play Blackjack.
The reason is simple.
With Craps, you have to stand up.
With Blackjack, you get to sit down.

But I decided to walk over to the table where Al
Michaels was playing Craps.
Because I had the line. (See my essay labeled "Beach,
The Nude").

I walked up to the pitboss, and asked "Where's the
main crap game?"
He said "What are you talking about?"
I said "I want to play at the main crap game. Where is
it?"
He said, "Sir, I don't know what you're talking about."
I was well-dressed enough to be called "Sir".
I said "Well, this can't be the main crap game. Al
Michaels is working it".
Al Michaels, good sport that he was, giggled.

Now, I'm 6 foot 5. And a lady who was about 4 foot
ten, standing directly in front of me, immediately
turned around, looked up at me and stared daggers.
She said "Al Michaels is a GREAT broadcaster. How
DARE you!"
I said "Lady, I agree with you. I think he's terrific. I'm
just making a joke!
She said "Don't 'Lady' me! I'm Al Michaels mother!
MRS. Michaels to you!"
I had not made a friend.
I skulked away, as quietly and quickly as I could, as Al
Michaels giggled longer and louder.

So when the Sands was blowed up, I considered it a
mercy-killing.
I'd also hoped it would help obliterate the Limeliters
experience and the Al Michaels experience from my
mind.

Apparently it hasn't.

*****

It's Not The Audience's Fault. It's Your Fault.

When Lowell Ganz and I were first hired to work on the "Odd Couple" writing staff, I learned a lot about myself that first week.

First, I felt very much out of place and insecure as a writer.
This is because when we wrote the spec script that got us hired, Lowell was very much the joke writer, and I was very much the storyteller and character writer.
Any jokes that I contributed to that script were essentially character jokes, and Lowell's were essentially one-line snappers.
And great ones.

And it became apparent early on to me that "The Odd Couple" was much more joke-oriented, one-line snapper-oriented, and less story and character joke-oriented.
It was a show that was dominated by punch-up writers. That was not me.
So I was very insecure.
My main contribution to that series, according to several who worked on it, including me, was the somewhat successful attempt to make the show more mature and reality based.
Garry Marshall used to refer to the kind of show I liked to write as "Internal Shows".
Shows about the real problems of two middle-aged Jewish divorced men, rather than cartoons about them going on "Let's Make A Deal" for no really good reason.

Shows about worrying about getting older, about legitimate problems they might have with their social lives, their fears, part-time parenting, etc.

I wasn't against sillyness, I just was always looking for ways to justify it legitimately.
But hanging over all of this was my insecurity about joke-writing.

However, one thing that I never was insecure about was an ability I knew I had from day one-----
an unwavering accuracy in my mind about what would and would not work in front of the live audience of 300 people.
I knew that if the second syllable in a word was accented rather than the first, it would get a laugh. Or vice-versa.
Or if you added an "a", or a "the", or a "but" to a sentence in the right place, it would guarantee a laugh.
Conversely, if you took out one of those words, it would kill the laugh.

I don't know how or why I can do that.
It is pure instinct.
But I have it.
And it has served me very well all these years.
It's the reason that I rarely if ever re-write my own material.
To me, if it's good enough to get from my ball-point pen to my yellow legal pad, it's good enough to show people.
And I've never been proven wrong.
It's one of the very few areas of my life that I have any confidence in, and I have every confidence in it.
This has led me to have absolute faith in the judgment of the 300 or so people comprising the live audience.
This applies to sitcom tapings and theatre.

If you're doing theatre in a smaller house, it's far less predictable. Any small bloc of people can influence the rest of the audience in an unexpected way.

But if you have at least 300 people, seated, facing the stage, who understand English, to me it's a no-brainer.
Pure instinct.

And they are always right.
If they don't respond the way you want them to, then you failed. Not them.

This instinct has usually provided me with a total joyousness as I'd leave my office and head down to the stage on show night.
I'd usually rub my hands together, smile, and think to myself "Boy, I can't wait for them to see this".
Whenever I felt this way, I was rewarded with a totally positive audience response.

But I didn't always feel this way.

There were times I knew I'd go down there knowing I'd fail.
On those nights, I'd invariably take my lumps.
Sometimes I just didn't have enough time to get it the way it needed to be.
Sometimes the network or studio or star took the bat out of my hands.
And we'd fail.
As I knew we would.
But it was never a mystery to me.
It was never "Gee, I wonder how they're going to react tonight?".
I always knew.
Because of my instinct, and the knowledge that the audience is always right.

Billy Wilder once said that as individuals, each and every person comprising the audience is an idiot. But collectively, they're a genius.

There was one night that I knew we would both succeed and fail.
Impossible you say?
Au contraire.

Telling this will be an education about how shows are created. Or in this case, co-created.

The show in question is "Laverne and Shirley".

Any time there is a media story about Garry Marshall, it usually begins "Garry Marshall, creator of 'Happy Days' and 'Laverne and Shirley'........"

This is an example of media sloppiness and laziness.

Those stories should read "Garry Marshall, creator of "Happy Days" and co-creator, with Lowell Ganz and Mark Rothman, of "Laverne and Shirley". That's the way it appears on the screen.

But that would require media neatness and alertness. This has consigned Lowell and me to being mere footnotes in TV history.

There was a network documentary about "Laverne and Shirley" where Garry was interviewed.

Lowell and I were never contacted, or mentioned.

Our names passed by very quickly in tiny letters along with a lot of other names in the end credits crawl.

When Garry was on screen, the graphic on the lower portion read "Garry Marshall, Creator". I complained to the Writer's Guild, to exact my pound of flesh from the makers of the documentary.

Those lazy, sloppy media thugs.
It went to arbitration.
I won the battle.
And lost the war.
They changed the graphic to "Garry Marshall, Co-Creator" for future airings.

Now, the last thing I wanted to do, or ever want to do, is bring down Garry.
Lowell and I both owe Garry a great deal.
All I wanted to do was raise us up to where I thought we legitimately belonged.

But with my readership continuing to grow in popularity, I now consider myself a member of the media.
And I'd like to be one of the few neat and alert ones.

So I'm going to lay out how "Laverne and Shirley" was created, step by step, as I remember it.

There is no good reason for anyone to object to this, except perhaps on the grounds that it may seem like sour grapes.
But people have bellyached about far less important things than this.
Bear in mind that this is my single most important Credit.
And nobody is out there to take care of it but me.
You can draw whatever conclusion you want. Or you can skip the rest of this completely.
It's up to you.
Any way you want to go, I won't be offended.

1) While working on "Happy Days", Lowell and I were invited to write an episode of a new MTM series called "Paul Sand in Friends and Lovers".

This came about because Penny Marshall was a regular in the cast, and recommended us to Jim Brooks and Allan Burns.
We wrote the episode.
Paul Sand played a cellist in the Boston Symphony.

We all worked out a story about how Paul was going through a cold streak in his dating life.

It built to a scene at the end where Paul, on the advice of his brother-in-law, goes to the supermarket to hit on women, and fails spectacularly.

2) They shoot the episode, and we attend the filming, only to see that the script was totally rewritten.
They got cold feet about portraying Paul as a loser this early in the series, and turned it into a show about Paul having to choose between two different women.
Only one of our scenes survived.
NOT the supermarket scene.
But we got paid, and received full writing credit.
MTM was a class act.

3) The show is cancelled after 11 episodes.
Penny is out of work.

4) Penny shows our "Paul Sand" script to Garry.

5) Garry, always looking out for his sister, has a brilliant idea.
He often had brilliant ideas.
He called us into his office and told us that he read our script, loved the supermarket scene, and suggested that it not go to waste.
We should do that scene on "Happy Days". Richie, at Fonzie's behest, would hit on women in the supermarket.
MTM apparently didn't mind.
Only the scene should be done in the first act.

Not the second.
The second act would be the result of his failure.
Fonzie sets the two of them up with blind dates.
A couple of Bimbos. Dirty Girls.
Garry had the Bimbos already picked out.
Penny Marshall and Cindy Williams.

6) We got paid to write a new script for "Happy Days",
incorporating all these concepts.

7) We write. We give these Bimbos names.
Lowell comes up with Laverne DeFazio for Penny.
I come up with Shirley Feeney for Cindy.

8) We shoot the episode. The 300 people told us it
was great. Something I already knew going in.

9) Garry did the thing that sold the series.
Something that Lowell and I could never do in a
million years:
Get Fred Silverman On The Phone.
Silverman ran ABC at the time.

Garry smelled a series.
He was great at smelling a series.

10) Fred Silverman loves what he sees, but has one
reservation.
Nowhere in this episode is there a scene with just
Laverne and Shirley, going one on one, talking to each
other.
He requests that a scene be shot that happens after
the blind date, at the girls' apartment, summing up
the evening, and their lives.

11) Garry tells us to go off and write this scene.
We do so, eagerly.

This scene required a lot of character exploration by Lowell and me before we could write.
We decided that they work in a brewery, as bottlecappers.
One is a dreamer, the other is a realist.
One wants to marry no less than a doctor, and the other would be happy with a sailor.

One was more dainty, one more rough around the edges.
None of this was indicated in the episode we'd already shot.

12) We run all this past Garry.
He approves. We start writing.
And we write.
And we write.
And we sculpt.
And we chisel.
And we hone.
And we've got gold.

Garry loves it, and we plan to shoot it as is.

13) Garry writes a treatment.
I don't remember if it had our names on it as well as his.
It really doesn't matter.
In it, he invents the character of Shirley's father as a regular.
We ended up doing one episode involving Shirley's father somewhere down the line.

He also invents Carmine Ragusa.
Pretty much as he ends up being.

By the third episode, they were no longer bimbos.
ABC was deservedly antsy about that.
Now, I'm notsaying, nor would I ever say that Lowell and I created this series and Garry didn't.

I'm just saying that we are entitled to more credit than we've been given over the years, and this has been the only opportunity I've ever had to express myself about it.

Okay. Enough tub-thumping.

14) We shoot the scene.

Oh. Did I mention that while we were writing and writing and sculpting and chiseling and honing to shoot this scene the following Friday, that we were still the Head Writers of "Happy Days", and that they were shooting that same Friday too?
On the same stage?
Before the Laverne and Shirley scene?
And that we never took care of business on "Happy Days" because of it?

We basically gave "Happy Days" a first draft to shoot that week.
What would you have done?
We were only hired hands on "Happy Days".

We were in on the ground floor of "Laverne and Shirley".
Our priorities were in order.

So Lowell and I walked down to stage 19 at Paramount that Friday night, knowing that we were going to fail and succeed.

We were embarrassed to look at the "Happy Days" cast as they went through their paces, with the audience actually becoming an oil painting.
They came out for their curtain calls.
To an extremely light smattering of applause.
This was unprecedented.
The cast loved us.
And we loved them.
And we had let them down.

For the first time.
They all looked at us, like a herd of wounded deer.
The audience couldn't wait to get out of there.

They started filing out during the curtain calls.
Unprecedented.

Garry, who had been doing the warmup all evening,
pleaded with the audience to re-take their seats.
"Folks, please stick around for a few more minutes.
We have a scene to show you from a new show. I think
you'll like it a lot."

Reluctantly, the audience sat back down.

We had redressed Fonzie's bedroom to look like
Laverne and Shirley's apartment.
It was screened off from the audience.
Penny and Cindy were seated at the kitchen table,
behind the screen.
The stage lights in that area were turned on.

Now, you must realize that the "Happy Days" episode
that introduced Laverne and Shirley hadn't aired yet.
Nobody in the audience knew who these girls were.
And Garry offered no explanation as to who they were.

The screens were pulled back.
The three cameras hit their marks. They started
rolling film.

Action.

Penny talks to Cindy.
Cindy talks to Penny.

Immediate pandemonium.

They laughed at EVERYTHING.

EV-VER-REE-THING!!!

The same 300 people.

The same oil painting.

They're always right.

Garry tacks the new scene on the end of the "Happy Days" episode, removing the first act.

(The supermarket scene. Remember?) It becomes the Laverne and Shirley presentation film.

Fred Silverman, also real good at smelling hits, immediately ordered a season's worth, and it was Number One from the get-go.

More irony: That episode of Happy Days we shot that night? It was about Arnold (Pat Morita) getting married.

When it aired, it became the first time "Happy Days" was Number One in the ratings.

And it held Number One until that first episode of "Laverne and Shirley" aired.

We all thought of adding a father for Laverne after we made the sale.

And Lenny and Squiggy, of course, came from the moon.

*****

No, Lenny and Squiggy Are Not Aliens.

I was being facetious.
There was facetiousness at work.

Lenny and Squiggy, in fact, did not come from the
Moon, or anywhere else in the outer galaxy.

A lot of interest has been expressed about how Lenny
and Squiggy landed on "Laverne and Shirley".
I think this will explain it:

Knowing Penny Marshall previously (She was, after
all, Myrna on the Odd Couple),
I attended several parties at her house.
This was when she was married to Rob Reiner.
Most members of hip show business were usually on
hand.
They were memorable evenings.

I remember one night when Albert Brooks was there,
holding court.
When you were in a room full of people that included
Albert Brooks, you never wanted to leave it:
1) Because you'd be afraid you'd miss something, and

2) Because as soon as you did, you knew you'd be
mocked by him behind your back.

Albert spent half the evening mocking Harry Shearer
to his face (Harry, a great wit and conversationalist,
just couldn't compete with Albert Brooks) and the
other half trying to convince everybody that
something called the Cleveland Wrecking Company
was the biggest of its kind in the world.
He had mentioned it in passing.
And he drew blanks from all in the room.

He went, perhaps mock, ballistic. You never really knew with him.

"You mean, you've never heard of the Cleveland Wrecking Company? It's the biggest!!!"
Nobody really questioned him, but that didn't stop him from satisfying his apparently obsessive need to prove that it, in fact, existed, and was in fact, the biggest.

He looked through the L.A. Yellow Pages, and saw a small ad for it.
This proved it existed, but certainly didn't prove that it was the biggest.

He then called long-distance information in Cleveland Ohio, asked for the number, and called it.

This being a Saturday Night, all he got was a recorded message, but on the message it said something like "You have reached the Cleveland Wrecking Company, the biggest name in wrecking".
He called the number repeatedly, each time putting the phone up to someone else's ear.

After several choruses of "We believe you, Albert!" He beamed, and said "I told you! The biggest!!"

One of the funniest things I have ever witnessed.

Also witnessing this were David Lander, Michael McKean, and the aforementioned Harry Shearer, who along with Christopher Guest, were members of a satirical comedy group called The Credibility Gap. Perhaps the hippest, funniest, best group of its kind ever assembled.
They were to satire what Miles Davis is to Jazz.

It was the first time I'd met them.

The Sunday after "Laverne and Shirley" sold, Penny
threw together a party at her house to celebrate.
Of course, Lowell Ganz and I attended.
We were already signed to produce the series, and had
a lot to say about how it was going to take shape.

During the party, Penny coaxed David Lander and
Michael McKean to get up and do a routine they
regularly performed for Credibility Gap audiences,
called "Lenny and Anthony".
Much more subtle names than Lenny and Squiggy.
I don't remember whose idea it was to eventually
right-wing it up and call them Lenny and Squiggy.
David and Michael bristled at it.
Lowell and I weren't thrilled about it.
That left several other suspects.
But, apparently for the sake of mass appeal, they
became Lenny and Squiggy.

So David and Michael go into their act as Lenny and
Anthony.

Funniest thing I've ever seen.

It left "The Cleveland Wrecking Company" in the dust.
The audience was hysterical.

Lowell and I quickly realize that the whole raison
d'etre for this party was for Penny to enable David and
Michael to audition for us.

We had only one concern: It was also the filthiest
thing we had ever seen.
Afterwards, Lowell and I talked it over.
I don't remember who said what, but the conversation
went something like:

"Whattya think?"

"I don't know."

"Do you think it works clean?"

"If it's one-fifth as funny clean as it is filthy, it's still as funny as anything that's been on TV."

"Let's do it".

So they became Lenny and Squiggy.
And were about one-fifth as funny as Lenny and Anthony.

This is no knock on Lenny and Squiggy.
America has already passed judgement on them.

But it's too bad America never got to see Lenny and Anthony.

I've often referred to "Laverne and Shirley" as a left-wing show in right-wing trappings.

Everyone involved in it was from the hip end of show business.
But it was all dressed up as a typical cornball sitcom.

Maybe that's why it was so popular.
It could be watched on two levels---the square, and the hip.

Alan Arkin used to show up in the audience at "Laverne and Shirley" filmings.
How's that for hip?

He loved Lenny and Squiggy.
He should have only seen Lenny and Anthony.

My ex-wife and I eventually bought Penny and Rob's house from them.
My only request, as part of the deal, was that they let me keep the telephone that Albert Brooks used to call the Cleveland Wrecking Company.

For my collection.

We moved in, and shortly thereafter, we nailed a plaque to the living room floor.
It commemorated the spot where my ass fell off from having it laughed off from watching Lenny and Anthony.

*****

That Was My Desire.

I'm going tell you a story about the casting of "Laverne and Shirley" that no one involved in the production of that show, or anyone else, has ever been aware of.

Because I've never told anybody about it before.

As most of you who are familiar with the series know, we cast the wonderful comedian Phil Foster as Laverne's father, Frank DeFazio.
We knew it would be a good idea to have an interesting actor to play Laverne's gruff father.
Someone, ideally, who would bring out Laverne's softer side, by being much tougher than she was.
Someone who had a certain earthy charm, too.

And most important, someone who was really funny.
He'd fit in nicely as the owner of the local hangout, the pizza parlor-bowling alley, the Pizza Bowl.
It would help give us a funny place to go outside of the girls' apartment, and their work.

Garry Marshall and I both had Phil Foster in mind.
Garry was always very loyal to comedians who helped him get started writing comedy.
Phil was one of those.

There were other powers-that-be that were more resistant to the notion.
And not without decent reason.

Garry and I both thought Phil had all the necessary qualities.
He certainly was interesting.

I think "interesting" is what differentiates a good actor from an ordinary one.

I know a former actor who has now carved a modest niche in other areas of show business who pontificates about how you're not really an actor unless you always know your lines inside and out, never miss your blocking, and always hit your marks.
I've seen this guy's work.
He claims to have always known his lines inside and out, never missed his blocking, and always hit his marks.   I'll take him at his word.
But that didn't prevent him from being continually, relentlessly boring whenever on stage and screen.
I'm pretty sure that's why he's a former actor.

Phil Foster never knew his lines, never knew his blocking, never hit his marks.
And he constantly mumbled. But he was relentlessly interesting.
To me, that's much more important.

Billy Wilder, describing working with Marilyn Monroe on a couple of great movies, acknowledged that she never knew her lines and never hit her marks.
He said "I've got an Aunt Minnie, who could come in here, know all her lines, and always hit her marks. But nobody would pay good money to see my Aunt Minnie. 'Cause she's not so interesting".

Jackie Gleason's idea of "Blocking" when he was shooting "The Honeymooners", was to tell the director "Just tell the guy on Camera One to point it at me, and follow me wherever I'm going."
And it didn't matter where he went, because he was INTERESTING.

Phil's mumbling was the cause of everyone else's misgivings.
It was a little daunting.

He had mumbled his way through an episode of the
Odd Couple, and I found it and him adorable, though
a little scary.

I knew Garry needed support on this one, and I
campaigned hard for Phil.
The others involved in the decision had pretty high
regard for my casting sense.
And there wasn't really a good second choice.

We saw some lulus along the way.
One was former Heavyweight contender Lou Nova,
who was once knocked out by Joe Louis.
He plowed through his audition with a grin on his
face, as if he owned the room.
But he had nary a clue about what he was doing, or
where he was, for that matter.
As if Joe had just punched him in the head.
And he was one of the finalists.

Phil was looking better and better.
I went to the mat for Phil. "I know he mumbles. We'll
make it work for us", I half-believed.

We signed him, and I think he was a major asset to
the show.

About a week and a half after we signed Phil, I was at
home, watching TV.
There was a rerun of an old episode of Make Room for
Daddy on, from the late 50's, starring Danny Thomas.
I used to watch that show every week when I was a
kid.
The guest on the show that night was Frankie Laine,
the great singer.

You know, "Mule Train", "That's My Desire",
"Jezebel". Frankie Laine.

He appeared as himself.
He was wonderful.
He had a lot of dialogue.

Funny, charming, enormous presence, Italian, like
Laverne, maybe not all that gruff, but INTERESTING.

In the mid 1970's, he was about the same age as Phil.
And he didn't mumble.
He wasn't doing all that much those days.
And he was a 50's icon.
"Laverne and Shirley" took place in the 50's.

He would've been great. We missed a bet.

Timing is everything.
If I'd seen that episode of Make Room For Daddy two
weeks prior, I would have yelled "Stop the Presses!"
no matter how much I'd campaigned for Phil Foster.
But the boat had sailed.
It was a done deal.
No point in even bringing it up.
So I never did.
Until now.

Getting Frankie Laine to play Laverne's father.

That was my desire.

My unrequited desire.

*****

The $500 Joke.

The younger you are when you work as a writer on a
TV series, the more, and the more profoundly, you get
your heart broken.
"The Odd Couple" was a show where everyone
involved pretty much cared passionately about what
they were doing.

I cared passionately about turning out good work.

Tony Randall, Jack Klugman, and Garry Marshall
cared passionately about doing good work.

Garry's father, Tony Marshall, who Garry had as one
of the Producers of "The Odd Couple", cared
passionately about saving money and not spending
money.
That was his job, and he was passionate about it.

Sometimes I was so in love with my script and my
heart got broken because Jack and Tony weren't, and
summarily rejected things in it.
And I was powerless to do anything about it.

Other times I was so in love with my script and my
heart got broken because Tony Marshall would pipe
up with his usual mantra:
"Do we really have to spend money on THIS?".
And then things that I loved would get summarily
rejected, on that basis.

The penultimate example of this was the episode
where Oscar and Felix were arrested for ticket
scalping.

This ended up in a courtroom, where Felix acted as
his own attorney.

We did one of these each year that I was there, and they remain some of my favorite episodes.

The premise here was that they were arrested for ticket scalping because Oscar tried to get a date, but struck out right and left.
So they were left with an extra ticket, that Felix tried to give away.
But it appeared that he was trying to scalp it.

In each courtroom show we did, we figured out a different and unique way for Felix to humiliate Oscar on the witness stand.
In one, Felix portrayed Oscar as a "Stooge of Management".
In another, he portrayed Oscar as a " Divorced, Degenerate Gambler".
In this one, he portrayed Oscar as "A Slob of a Loser who Can't Get a Date".

And, of course, Felix always expected Oscar to be grateful afterwards.

Well, we did effect this particular humiliation upon Oscar in this episode.
But we had written something that really would have been icing on the cake.
While Felix had Oscar on the witness stand, he got Oscar to admit that after trying really hard, he couldn't get any woman, of all the women he knew, (and some strangers) to go to this Broadway Show with him that they had tickets for.

Then, in our script, Felix turned to the gallery and requested that all the women present that Oscar Madison asked out that particular evening please rise.

A motley collection of women, all sizes and shapes, would then rise, check each other out, then stare at Oscar, heightening his humiliation to the fifth power.

That element was dashed by the end of the first reading.

We heard the usual mantra:
"Do we really have to spend money on this?
It's at least eleven extras.
It's a five hundred dollar joke.
Is it really worth $500?"

We thought it was. We were quickly outvoted. It was gone.

The show was still really good, but this would have made it great.
I suppose I could have offered to pony up the $500 myself, but I wasn't in that kind of position financially, and I knew it would set a terrible precedent.
It would have been "You want the joke that badly, come up with $500."

It still left a bitter taste in my mouth, knowing that for the lack of $500, a great sight gag was lost.

Nine years later, I was the show runner on "The New Odd Couple", with Ron Glass and Demond Wilson as Felix and Oscar, respectively.

The orders came down from the network and the studio to recycle the original scripts we did on the original Odd Couple series.
I didn't mind this. There are remakes in movies all the time.

Why not remakes for TV?

So I chose what were basically my favorites to remake.
My first choice was the ticket scalping show.
I had a built-in axe to grind.

I was going to restore that moment that never made it past the first reading the first time around.
I was going to prove that the joke was worth at least $500.
Although, by now, with inflation and all, it was going to cost more like $1100.
I thought it was worth at least $1100.

And now, there was nobody there to say "Do we really have to spend money on THIS?"

And at this point, if I had to, I was doing well enough financially that I would have ponied up the dough myself.
But it never came to that.

So we hired the eleven female extras.
And we did the eleven hundred dollar joke.

And the live audience gave it the biggest laugh you can possibly imagine.

I was vindicated.
Nine years later.

Thomas Wolfe was wrong.

You CAN go home again.

*****

The Names Have Been Changed To Protect The Innocent.

"The Story You Are About To See Is True.
The Names Have Been Changed To Protect The Innocent."

These were the opening words of every episode of the series "Dragnet".

My ex-wife used to love to watch "Dragnet" when she was a little girl.

But it was on past her bedtime.

Going into the last commercial, the announcer would always say "The results of this case in just a moment".

My ex-wife's parents watched "Dragnet", and unbeknownst to them, their little daughter would be sitting on the staircase landing, watching along with them.
Once, during the last commercial, she was spotted on the landing and immediately ordered to be off to bed.
And she cried out "Can't I just see the zults?
I just wanna stay up to see the zults!!"

After she told me this story, the word "results" was never used in our house.
It forever became "zults"

Do you know what a "Roman-a-clef" is?

Here's the definition, according to Wikipedia:

A roman à clef or roman à clé (French for "novel with a key") is a novel describing real life, behind a façade of fiction.

The 'key' is usually a famous figure or, in some cases, the author.
Well, this is going to be an Essay-a-clef.

Ordinarily, I hate using this form.
I've been totally candid about everything so far, but in this case we must protect the innocent.
And one of the characters is SO innocent that I don't want to hurt him.
And one of the characters is so guilty that I don't want to get sued.

Years ago, I wrote, produced, and directed one of my plays, a romantic comedy,
in Los Angeles in one of those 100 seat Equity Waiver Theaters that dot the L.A. landscape.

Equity Waiver means you don't have to pay the actors.

There's something you should know about theater in L.A:
Nobody goes to see it.

I mean, they'll go to the Dorothy Chandler, or the Mark Taper Forum, or the Ahmanson downtown.
But they don't go to the Equity Waiver Theaters in any kind of serious numbers.

So why are productions done there?
Two reasons.
Either to serve as gymnasiums for actors, places for them to work out.
Or to serve as Showcases for actors, directors, or writers with Agendas.

I put my play in one of those theaters because of my Agenda.
I wanted to demonstrate to Show Business that I wasn't just a sit-com guy, but a real playwright and theater director.

(And maybe they'd also see this play as a Back-Door Pilot.)

Heavy Agenda.

Very important TV stars are sometimes willing to work in Equity Waiver Theater, for free, because they have Agendas.
One such important TV star, a veteran leading actress of several TV series and too many TV-Movies to count, clamored to be the female lead in my play.
For free.
Because she had an Agenda.
She wanted to prove to the industry that she was adept at comedy.
Comedy was something she was rarely considered for.
She was willing to read for me.
She had the tools for comedy.
And her name value would certainly fill some seats.
So I wanted her.
Let's call her "Millie".
But Millie's agent was very protective of Millie.
Let's call him "Asshole".
That's what most agents are called anyway.
Asshole wanted to make sure that the leading man would be someone of her stature, and would make her look good.
This was a tall order to fill, trying to find someone like that who'd work for free.
But we all started to compile lists of potential leading men who would fill the bill.
We would contact the actors Millie deemed acceptable.
We had a few solid nibbles, but couldn't nail anyone down.

The closest I came was a major comedian who got big around the same time as Robert Klein and George Carlin.

He was more mainstream, had had a short-lived sitcom, and was just itching to have another go at it. Let's call him "Dick", although he certainly wasn't one.

Dick's big plaint was how he opened the doors for guys like Seinfeld who had these huge hit sitcoms, but he has no respect as an actor, and couldn't get another series.
I'd seen him complain about this on TV.
Meanwhile, he was making money hand-over-fist in Vegas, and nightclubs, and concerts.
So he saw my play, which he loved, as an opportunity to get that respect.
He read for me and was really good.
But he was wavering.
It would mean giving up a lot of money.

I told him a story I had heard, about Mel Torme.
Mel Torme was offered the opportunity to play Mickey Rooney's brother on what turned out to be an Emmy award winning episode of "Playhouse 90", written by Rod Serling in the late 50's.
Mel Torme was torn.
He moaned to his friend Edmond O'Brien, who was already cast in another part in this episode, about how he was only being offered $500 to do the show, and how it would mean turning down the $5000 a week for three weeks he would have earned in nightclubs. O'Brien said to him, "Melvin, you should be paying them."

Torme played Mickey Rooney's brother, and was great.

I told Dick that story.
He understood.
I almost had him.
But in the end, he couldn't turn down the money.

Next case.

I considered Casting my forte, and my gut usually proved right.

Starting to scramble, a name entered my head that I thought would be really good.
The star of a MAJOR action series in the 60's, who I had seen be VERY funny.
Let's call him "Manny".
Manny wasn't all that visible lately, and I had a feeling doing this play with Millie might do him some good, get him great exposure and that he'd do it for free.

Manny didn't even make it to Millie's ears.
I mentioned Manny to Asshole, who said "Him?
Are you crazy?! He's not funny! And he's got to be a hundred years old!
You're not going to put him on the same stage with my Millie!!
That's how he thought, and that's how he talked.
He was wrong, but I wasn't going to press the matter.

I later learned that Asshole not only represented Millie.
He also represented Manny.

How would you like to be Manny, having Asshole as your agent?
Or at least this particular Asshole.

So we pressed on.
The longer it took, the fewer qualifications were insisted on.

Stature became less important than making Millie look good.

So I thought of really good actors I'd worked with, and mentioned someone primarily known as a comedian, very well-known in the 60's and 70's.
This was the 90's.

Millie and Asshole deemed him acceptable.
Let's call him "Jackie" (What else is new?).

In the interim, I was coaching Millie on how to be better in the part, even though the play wasn't completely cast yet.

After a couple of sessions, I get a call from Asshole: "Millie really thinks a lot of you. She's reading for a sitcom pilot next week. Would you be willing to give up your Sunday and go to Millie's house to coach her for her audition? I'd really owe you for this".

I agreed.

Like I said, Millie had the tools, and was very malleable.   She completely trusted me.

It was good material, which made it easier.
I made many suggestions, which she immediately adapted to easily.
By the time we were done, I thought she was quite good.

For whatever reason, she wasn't cast.
But I felt redeemed when the pilot, which didn't sell, was aired the following summer.
The actress who was cast, let's call her "Swoosie", played it exactly as I had instructed Millie to play it.
And was quite good.

Okay. So I call Jackie's agent, and explained the situation.
He requested a script.
I shortly hear from Jackie.
He loves it and wants to do it.
Raving and raving about the script.
And he's thrilled that Millie wants to work with him.
Jackie is in.

I meet Jackie for lunch.
He has bandages on his face.
He's just had a facelift.
He tells me he had it done live on the Internet.
So he could get it done for free.

A week later, we hold the first cast reading at Millie's house.
Jackie is terrific.
Millie seems to be keeping her distance.
I sense Trouble In River City.

Everyone leaves.
I ask Millie if anything is wrong.
"No, everything's fine".
I less than believe her.
I leave, with the citizens of River City yelling "Trouble! Trouble! Trouble!" in my car.

Next day, I get a call from Asshole.
"Millie can't do the play. She's really sorry". I thought this was probably not a good time to mention to Asshole that he owes me.

Turns out, between the time she accepted Jackie until the first cast reading, she found out about Jackie's free Internet facelift.
She couldn't get past the words "Tacky" and "Cheesy".
I really couldn't blame her.

So I had Jackie and no Millie.
And now Jackie is threatening to pull out if don't get someone of equal stature to Millie.

I tried.
But there were several actresses of that stature who also thought Jackie represented "Tacky" and Cheesy".
Jackie was sensational in the part and I really didn't want to lose him.
And I thought he might still be a bit of a draw.

The best I could do was a really terrific actress and comedienne who I knew, very well-known for her only TV series, a big hit show, now considered legendary.
But I think it typecast her.
She thinks so too.
People had trouble thinking of her as anybody else.
This happens sometimes.
As Garry Marshall was often given to say, "It's not a fair business".
Let's call her "Aurora".

Jackie didn't want to hear about Aurora.
His almost precise words were "Don't give me no Aurora!"
I said "What happened to the raving and raving about the play?"
He said, "That's when you had Millie!"

I loved and love Aurora.
Personally and professionally.

So here's the Zults:

I told Jackie to go screw. I was going with Aurora.

I was going with less star power.
For the male lead, I went with an actor whose work I loved, but who was only known in more limited circles.
He was actually much better known as a child actor.
Let's call him "Morris".

Aurora, matched up romantically with Morris?

Well, Morris was now 50. It worked great.

It was wonderful to watch the two of them together.

We got great reviews, and Equity Waiver being what it was, did sparse business.

Morris left during the run. We got someone else.
A really good actor, with no drawing power.

My lips are sealed as to who all of these people are.
You'd have to know me really well to get that kind of
information out of me.
If you think you know, keep it to yourself.
I didn't do it this way to tease you.
It was the only way I felt I could tell this story with
any kind of tact.

You know what? After Morris left the run, I probably
should have gone after Manny.
He still would have been great.

And Asshole still owed me one.

He still does.

*****

Joyce DeWitt: She Was Almost The Sheriff.

Okay. I'm sitting in my house in the Midwest in 1986, and I get a call from an executive from Lorimar, the TV and Movie studio in L.A.
I'd worked with this executive before.
She was a liaison for ABC when I was the show-runner for "New Odd CUPPle".

They had shot one without me, which sucked.
Then they brought me in with someone else to take over.
It then became very good in their eyes and mine.
Then, through rather unfortunate circumstances, after about ten episodes, I quit.
The someone else stayed, and they hired two other people to replace me.
This has become somewhat standard procedure:
I leave, and they hire two people to replace me.
He said, immodestly.
Then, in everybody's eyes, it sucked again.

Cut to: four years later. This ABC liaison had now become head of Comedy Development for Lorimar.
She apparently put two and two together, and it came to four.

The NBC owned-and operated stations, known in the "biz" as the "O and O's", of which there were five: New York, Chicago, Los Angeles, Washington, and I think, San Francisco, decided that they were going to attempt to single-handedly knock off "Wheel of Fortune".
You can see how successful that effort was.

But they plowed ahead, and concocted a formula and an ad campaign called "Prime Time Begins at 7:30".

If you lived in any of these cities, you might vaguely recall this.

The idea was to put a new sitcom each night of the Monday through Friday week.
These were essentially syndicated sitcoms, which, in the other cities, would be on any old time.

Lorimar desperately wanted to become part of "Prime Time Begins At 7:30".
So they carefully examined their shelves of unsold pilots and came up with this show that they had shot five years previously.
About a lady sheriff.
It starred someone named Caroline McWilliams, whom you might recall from "Benson". I didn't.

The NBC O and O guy insisted that what was needed for this show to be given a berth on "Prime Time Begins at 7:30 was a Star bigger than Caroline McWilliams, and an experienced show runner.
I apparently was considered the latter.
And my name showed up on a short list of show runners who might be available.
The Head of Comedy Development, her math skills still good, contacted me to see if I was interested, and sent me a tape of this previously made pilot.

I watched it.
It was far from the worst thing I've ever seen.
It was far from the best thing I've ever seen.
But it seemed eminently fixable, and if the fixes were made, could be fun to work on, and actually have some integrity.

So I called back Lorimar and enumerated my problems, which I referred to, at least to myself, as my fourteen points (an homage to Woodrow Wilson. I'm sure he would have been proud.):

1- This woman was a divorcee, a political appointment, with no background in law enforcement, not needing the money.
In order to take this job, she had to leave her two young children with her fifteen year old, which seemed rather irresponsible.

2- She should have earned this job by having a background in law enforcement.
For more sympathy, she should have been a widow.

3- She should have needed the money.

4- She should have had someone more responsible to raise the kids while she was out Sheriffing.

5- We needed a funny reason to go home.
Having the Sheriff's funny mother living in the house to take care of the kids, to me solved all of these problems.
I had Pat Carroll in the back of my mind.

6- The main set was absolutely dysfunctional.
It was a hallway, with a receptionist, leading to other offices.
I couldn't picture much action taking place there.
Barney Miller had it right: A group of desks for the officers, and a jail cell in the background for the funny prisoners to shout things through.

7- It took place in Indiana. Hardly fascinating.
How about someplace a little more exotic, like Lake Tahoe?
It would be more conducive for Show Business guest stars to show up naturally, what with all the showrooms in the casinos.

Not like The Patty Duke Show, where they contrived
having guest stars show up because their cars would
break down in front of Patty's house in Brooklyn.
Something that happened all the time.

I could and have gone on and on.

I related all of my fourteen points to Lorimar.
They bought into everything I was saying.

Then they started picking my brain about casting
ideas.
I tossed out names like Lucie Arnaz, and Erin Grey,
from "Silver Spoons".
They asked me what I thought of Joyce DeWitt.
Not having seen "Three's Company" too often, not
being a fan of it, for reasons you will shortly hear
about, but enough to realize that she was probably the
weakest link, I had a rather tepid response.
They then asked me about Priscilla Barnes, who
replaced Suzanne Somers on "Three's Company"
I certainly never made it that far to ever see Priscilla
Barnes, so I pleaded complete ignorance.

I was soon flown out to L.A. for a meeting, the point of
which was never made clear to me.
I got there and found myself in a large boardroom,
with everyone from Lorimar, and the head of the NBC
O and O's.
He was armed with "research"
He expressed his reservations about the pilot he saw.
They coincided with all of my reservations.
Only I had the solutions.
He loved all of my solutions.
He was ready to hand Lorimar one of the slots.
But we still needed a star.
He expressed his "research".
Apparently, the person America wanted to see in this
part was: Joyce DeWitt.

My heart sank momentarily, but quickly made the mental transition that we could surround her with funny people that she could essentially play straight to.

The meeting ended with much optimism.

Whenever I went from anywhere to L.A., I would usually stop off in Las Vegas for a few days beforehand, and on my way out, stop off in Las Vegas for a few days on my way back.

This was my plan here.

The Lorimar folks cautioned me not to go all the way home.

I might be needed again momentarily.

So I was primed to return to L.A. quickly.

At this point, I thought it behooved me to become more familiar with Joyce DeWitt's work.

So every night at 6:30, the local Vegas channel was showing reruns of "Three's Company" which were available for me to slog through.

I did. I wasn't any more impressed.

But these were the episodes that contained Priscilla Barnes.

I found myself being very impressed with her work, considering that she was basically slogging through sewage.

I called Lorimar, and expressed this opinion, saying that for whatever it was worth, and I'd thought it wasn't worth much at this point, that I thought Priscilla Barnes was terrific.

I was soon re-summoned to L.A.

Same boardroom. Same cast of characters.

Except instead of the O and O guy, there was Joyce DeWitt.

She was a lot better looking than he was.

She was a lot better looking than a lot of people.

I thought she looked a lot better in person than she did on TV.
I was in the process of extricating myself from a marriage, so she looked even better than that.

The Lorimar staff went into wooing overdrive in her direction.

"We love you".
"You're our first choice. You're our second choice. You're our third choice"
"You name it, that's what choice you are!"
"You can make a lot of money from this show".
"You'll share in the profits"
"Ownership! You'll have ownership!"
"We make movies here. We can put you in movies. Wouldn't you like to be in movies?!"

They were doing some good wooing.
And she was not unmoved.

But she had the same reservations about the pilot that she saw as I had, and the NBC O and O guy had.

They turned the floor over to me.
Recognizing my already established role as the Closer, I launched into my fourteen points.

By about the eighth point, I knew I had her.
She was looking at me the way a 40's bobby-soxer must have looked at Sinatra.

At this point, I was developing serious but unexpressed designs about getting into her pants.
So maybe she ain't all that funny.
I'll put funny people around her.
This show can work with her.
That's what went on in my mind at least.

I got done, and it was Hats In The Air Time.
They were practically carrying me around the room.

But she didn't commit in the room.

This was a Friday, and she said "Let me have the
weekend to think it over. I need to go on retreat".
Uh oh. This is someone who needs to go on retreat.
Sometimes it only takes a sentence like that to want to
leave her pants unsullied.
She started talking "cosmically".

So we had to wait the weekend.
Her on retreat. Dealing with the cosmos.
Me back in Vegas, with instructions not to go back
home until the deal was closed.

I figured I'd hear from them on Monday.
Nothing.
Tuesday.
Nothing.
Wednesday.
Nothing.
I was having serious trouble believing it.
I gave the performance of my life.
So did the Lorimar staff.
What the hell happened on retreat?
Thursday.
Nothing.
Friday. I hear from Lorimar."Well, we got her".
"Yeah?" I say.
"We got Priscilla Barnes".
"Huh?" I say.

Turns out that on Monday, Joyce DeWitt informs
them that her retreat went very well, and indeed she
was theirs.

In the interim, however, Lorimar checked with the
NBC O and O guy about the acceptability of Priscilla
Barnes.

And he apparently said "If she's okay with Mark, she's okay with me".
I had no idea I had that kind of influence.

So when Joyce DeWitt informed them that she was indeed theirs, they informed her that it was all well and good, but the money won't be all that wonderful as was discussed, and there won't be any sharing of profits.
No ownership.
And being put in movies will just be a rumor.
And that, if necessary, there are other choices.

They had cut a conditional deal with Priscilla Barnes that got her for two choruses.
Not even an entire song.

Joyce DeWitt declined this slap in the face, and was out.
And Priscilla Barnes was in.

No series for Joyce DeWitt since.
If only she hadn't gone on retreat.
Worlds might have turned, and you might not be seeing her mugshot all over the Enquirer.

*****

Priscilla Barnes: She Was Also Almost The Sheriff.

"We've got Priscilla Barnes", Lorimar told me.
Basically on my say-so.
She and Joyce DeWitt were friends, and miraculously,
wresting her part away from her did not affect their
friendship.

I first met Priscilla Barnes in New York.
A press conference was set up to announce the
beginning of "She's The Sheriff", as it was being
called, because that's what I decided to call it, (with no
objections) and to introduce Priscilla Barnes in her
return to regular weekly TV.
Her co-star, George Wyner, a survivor of the original
pilot, was introduced as well.
I had some script material prepared, and Priscilla and
George were going to act it out for the press.
I rehearsed it with them.
Priscilla had read the material, liked it, and said (her
first words to me) "Okay, I can do it this way, this way,
this way, this way, this way or this way. Pick one."
She then proceeded to demonstrate.
Every way was wonderful.
It was an embarrassment of riches.
My original instincts about her were right on the
money.

There is something very sexually arousing about
talent.
Not that I needed much coaxing.

The same is true about confident, aggressive women.
She was getting to me quickly.
Not that she gave a crap.

She informed me that she was treated very badly on
"Three's Company", and didn't want to have to go
through that again.
What she specifically didn't want to have to do on this
new show was to be the one who had to "lay the pipe".
This is a term I first heard from Garry Marshall.
He might have coined it.
It means spelling out the exposition of the story for
the audience.
It's usually a very dreary job for an actor to have to
"lay the pipe".

On "Three's Company", she was always relegated to
laying the pipe, and wanted none of it.
Neither Jack Klugman nor Tony Randall ever wanted
to lay the pipe.
They always wanted Al Molinaro or Penny Marshall to
do it.
But sometimes they weren't in the show that week,
and SOMEBODY had to lay the pipe.
Garry once told them, mockingly, "Maybe we can drag
a guy in off of Melrose Avenue and HE can lay the
pipe".
I saw Priscilla's point, but could make no promises
that I could be sure I'd keep.
I said I'd do what I could to keep the pipe out of her
hands as much as possible.
This response didn't seem good enough for her.

She and George acted out the scene, and were
wonderful.
The press seemed very responsive.

Things took longer than they were supposed to, and
I'd missed my flight back to the Midwest.
I was staying in New York overnight, as was Priscilla.

Someone from Lorimar suggested that we might like
tickets for a Broadway Show that night.

They arranged for house seats for "The Mystery of Edwin Drood", a clever musical whodunit that had a gimmick: the audience, by voting, would determine who, in fact dunit.
The actors were prepared to play out many different scenarios, depending on the audience's whim.
The show's lead actor, George Rose, was also its narrator.
He opened the show, explaining to the audience what they were in for, and how they were to participate, in a rousing opening number called "There You Are".
A real rouser, and Rose did it with incredible gusto.
He and the cast concluded it to wild, enthusiastic applause from the audience, during which, I turned to Priscilla and said "Now THERE'S a man who likes to lay the pipe".

And she scowled.

That's when I first sensed there would be trouble.

The press did its job. Priscilla made the cover of the Enquirer, with others returning to weekly TV.
The picture was actually flattering.

The second time I sensed there would be trouble was when she invited me to her acting class, for an evening of scenes, acted out by the students, in which she was to participate in one of.
(Is that English? Oh, well)
She did a knockout comedic version of Martha in "Who's Afraid of Virginia Woolf", in which she literally channeled Lucille Ball. She was brilliant.
I told her she was brilliant. But I also made the mistake of waxing ecstatic over another actress in another scene, and I never heard the end of it. In her mind, I wasn't there to look at no other actress in no other scene.

I guess it never occurred to Priscilla that the reason she got the part in "Sheriff" was because I wanted her. Who knows?

The third time was the charm.
Priscilla had some apparently mistaken notion that her deal provided her with some sort of guaranteed creative control.
The Lorimar people told me that she was essentially off her rocker on this one.
And this would have had to be something they would at least run by me, and they hadn't.

She and I had gone to a popular Chinese restaurant in L.A. that I had introduced her to.
She fell in love with it.

A few weeks later, I was in that restaurant with one of the writers, and we were going over a couple of scripts.
She shows up, to pick up a take-out order.
She sees us sitting there, working.
She wants to see the material.

Usually, I'm quite open to input from just about anybody.
Particularly someone as creative as she is.
But I've always made it a rule not to show material to anyone if I don't think it's ready to be shown.
And these scripts were not ready to be shown.
I told her this. She was not satisfied..
She bellowed something about creative control, got up, and stormed out of the restaurant, dragging her sack of Chinese food behind her.

And that was the last I saw of Priscilla Barnes.
It's a shame. She could have been great.
Also, no TV series since.
*****

How Priscilla Barnes Turned Into Suzanne Somers.

The next thing I heard after Priscilla Barnes stormed out of the Chinese restaurant was from the Lorimar execs.

Priscilla had presented them with an ultimatum: Either she has the "creative control" she was "Guaranteed", or she was walking.

After they all stopped giggling, they and I considered all the options.

They could sue her brains out, and/or they could get someone more preferable.

They considered themselves in the catbird seat.

They were loving this.

They basically asked themselves the musical question "Who in the wide world would we like to play this part?"

What I hadn't been privy to was that before I was part of the package, they had already made overtures to Suzanne Somers, who had turned them down .

This was because it was still "Pilot Season" for the networks.
"Sheriff" was a syndicated show.
Several cuts below a network show.

She was holding out for a possible network pilot.
None had materialized.
Pilot season was now over.
Suzanne Somers was suddenly available.

She'd cost more, but would be worth it, because of all the extra stations she'd most-likely attract.

I had a major rooting interest at this point.
I wanted them to get Suzanne Somers.

I had some ownership in this show, and if it was a hit,
I'd do much better for myself.

I had no idea if she was any good, but I knew she
wasn't any worse than Joyce DeWitt.

We met with Suzanne and her husband, Alan Hamel,
who was her husband personally and professionally.

I can and have written volumes about this concept.
So have others.

I had one point that I had to get across---in order for
this show to work, she could not, in any way, shape or
form, play this part as she played Chrissie on
"Three's Company".

She'd have to play an intelligent adult, which is in fact
what she was, except perhaps as far as her choice in
husbands went.

If she played a stupid Sheriff, the show has no reality
base, and could not possibly work.

It can't be "Lucy becomes the Sheriff".

They both seemed to understand and accept this.

All you science buffs out there understand the usual
pecking order of the nether regions of existence.
From the top down: paramecium, celebrities'
husbands, and amoebae.

Alan Hamel had essentially driven Suzanne's career
off a cliff with his ill-fated attempt to renegotiate her
contract with "Three's Company"
He was Thelma. She was Louise.

I'll let you all make your own judgments about how "usual" celebrities husbands are in the vast scheme of things.

As a result of his actions, Suzanne was forced to prove that she would "behave herself" here.
So they required her to audition.

None of the parties involved had any doubts that she would pass, no matter how good or bad she was.
All she had to do was jump through the hoops they provided for her.

She swallowed whatever pride she had, and agreed to this.

So I went to her house on Venice Beach, armed with audition material, and we went over it.
I could see that she was missing some things.

I stopped the proceedings, looked her in the eyes and said "You don't know me very well, and there's no reason you should believe what I'm about to say, but here goes: I'm always right.
Oh, I've certainly made more than my share of mistakes in life. But not creatively.
Just do this the way I tell you, and you'll have no trouble getting through this.
Just climb on my back, and I'll get you across the finish line in grand style."

She, of course, looked at me as if I had three heads.
But for some reason, she was willing to buy in to this.

I honestly believed what I was saying. I still do.
Call it ego if you want.

I call it the result of my actual experience. And it has always served me very well.

She and I did the audition together, and she was just dandy.
She was aboard.

We'd shot about half-a-dozen episodes, each in front of a live audience, and we always got complete affirmation from them.
I had no doubt that we would.

But almost every week, during rehearsal, I'd receive the phone call that there was some crisis on the set, and I had to come down there and put out the fire.
This never disturbed me, because I've never handed a script to an actor that I wasn't convinced would work.

My attitude on those strolls down to the set was always "All right. What are they missing this time?"
I'd get down there, they'd show me their "problem", and I'd always say something like "Yeah, but if you do this, this, this, this, and this, the problem goes away"

So they'd do this, this, this, this, and this, and the problem would somehow always magically go away.

After six weeks of this, and the last time it happened, she looked up at me and said "Son of a bitch! You ARE always right!"

And from that moment on, we got along just famously.

Except once.

*****

Turning Suzanne Into Lucy.

After we shot the first seven shows, we had a week off.
This enabled Suzanne to have the opportunity to
headline at the Desert Inn in Las Vegas.

She was kind enough to invite all who wished to make
the trek to come to see her show as her guests.
Many of us did, including me.
I never needed much of an excuse to go to Vegas
anyway, and this certainly qualified as "not much of
an excuse".

I was actually quite curious to see what exactly it was
she did onstage that justified her being a headliner.
Was it that dexterity she had telling jokes?
Was it that certain way she had with a song?
Was it that dazzling display of terpsichory (dancing)
she'd put on?

None of the above.
Suzanne was simply a pre-packaged "personality".
That she was turned into a headliner was probably her
husband's most astounding accomplishment.

She kibitzed with the audience, told some half-assed
jokes, attempted to sing, did a few dance steps with
her "boys" backing her up, and this constituted
"headlining".

We were all sitting rather close to the stage, which
gave me the opportunity to turn around several times
and see how this was going over with the paying
public.

I saw a lot of dour faces.
Particularly from the men, whom you'd figure to be
her target audience.

With a show like this it's difficult to determine if the husbands dragged the wives to it, or the wives dragged the husbands.
But you just knew somebody dragged somebody.

The audience's reaction in general was rather tepid.

The Smothers Brothers were her opening act, and they were great, as usual.
They most-likely smarted from the undemocratic nature of the business that required them to open for her, instead of the other way around.
And the audience loved them.
If I were in Vegas, and not invited to the show, I might have gone anyway, just to see the Smothers Brothers.

The show ended, and we all trouped backstage to thank Suzanne, and tell her how wonderful she was.
This is what you have to do sometimes.

Later that night, I received a call from from Suzanne, inviting me to have lunch with her and Alan out at their home in the desert, about a half-hour out of town.
I said "Fine".
This is what you have to do sometimes.

All the way out there in the car, I was dreading it.
The citizens of River City were already chanting "Trouble! Trouble! Trouble!" in my ear.

Why the hell do they want me out there to have lunch with them?
What do they want?
Do they want me to punch up her act?
It sure needed it.
I hoped for the best.
It was not forthcoming.

I got there, and we had lunch.

Pretty soon into it, it turned into Lunch and Pummeling.

They weren't happy with the show.
Not her Desert Inn show.
"She's The Sheriff".

They had no good reason not to be happy with the show.
It was getting very good ratings, the live audience loved it, and loved her.

I pointed this out, but apparently I was missing the point.
She wanted to be Lucy.
You know.
The one thing I'd told her she couldn't be for this show to work, and she agreed to not being.
Of course, when I told her this, she had no power.
Now she did.
The show was an established success, with her in it.
This unlevels the playing field.

So, over very good Mexican food, they worked me over for what seemed like hours to agree to write an episode where she could be Lucy.

What it really boiled down to was that she felt she wasn't getting her fair share of the laughs in the show.
That everyone else was. Not her.
Not exactly the "Jack Benny generosity to the rest of the cast" approach to things.
I pointed out that what she said might be true, but look at what she is getting: acceptance as an adult.
Something she never had before.
This was worth something.
She didn't care.

She wanted to be Lucy.

I told them how much this went against my grain, and
how it might be something we couldn't recover from,
and I honestly didn't know if I could pull it off
successfully.
Maybe they needed someone else to run the show.

I ate those words almost as quickly as they left my
mouth, because I knew how disposable I had become.
Sure, I'd sold the series for Lorimar and put it on the
map for them, but that was old business.
At this point, I was the only one who cared about the
quality of the show, which I thought it had a
considerable amount of.
Once a show is established, the studio and network
people are really just shmatta salesmen.
Just cut the goods, and push the goods.
It doesn't really matter how good the goods are.
Oh, they'll give you notes up the wazzoo, but that's
just to justify their jobs.

So if Suzanne wanted to be Lucy, it would be fine with
them.
See, I harbored the quaint notion that a show, any
show, should cling to any integrity it could muster up.

I suppose this seems odd, considering that my track
record consisted of working on shows where integrity
was not the strong suit:
The Odd Couple, where it was "Anything for a joke".
Happy Days, which bore extremely little resemblance
to the period in which it was set, and once introduced
a Martian to spin off.
It also had a noted incident where someone who was
never on water skis before kept his leather jacket and
his boots on and jumped over a shark successfully.
Laverne and Shirley, where two of the characters
actually WERE from Mars.

But in all these instances, I was always the one who clung the most steadfastly to reason.
I usually went down fighting.

I always worked better when there was a strong reality underpinning, and I thought it was going to be a tough enough sell for Suzanne Somers to do this part convincingly without the excess baggage of her also doing it like an idiot.

Suzanne and Alan acquiesced. She would do the part intelligently.
She wouldn't try to be Lucy.

Until we had shot about six episodes.
By then, they had the power, and I lost it.
If it was a matter of replacing anyone, it would be me and not her.
I was expendable. Not her.

So after an afternoon of lunch and pummeling at their house in Las Vegas, they twisted my arm until I yelled "Uncle", and I agreed to write an episode where she could be Lucy.

I don't know what you all think of Lucy.
I know what I think.
I think that in her prime, during "I Love Lucy", she was unmatched.
Nobody could touch her.
The best comedienne of her generation, by far.
No contest.

That Suzanne, that ANYONE thought they could attempt to duplicate what she did and not look pale by comparison is ludicrous.
Suzanne didn't have those kind of comedic chops, and she wasn't a particularly physical performer.
So not only was it a bad idea for the show, it was a bad idea for her to try to pull off.

But the gun was put to my head, and Lorimar was standing by as the firing squad if necessary.

I don't know what you all think of "I Love Lucy".
I know what I think.
I think it was great.
About a third of the time.

I think it was okay.
About a third of the time.

I think it was downright annoying .
About a third of the time.

To me, it was annoying when it was all about arbitrary scheming.
When it was about "Let's get dressed up in gorilla suits so Ricky and Fred will buy us those new dresses we want."

It was okay when it was about Lucy scheming to get into show business.
At least it wasn't arbitrary.

It was great when Lucy was a victim of circumstance.
When she didn't drive the craziness.
When the craziness drove her.

When she accidentally got the trophy stuck on her head.

When she used too much yeast in the bread, and the bread flew out of the oven and across the kitchen, pinning her to the wall.

When she got stuck in the freezer.

When she got looped on Vita-Meata-Vegamin.

When they were traveling across the country and got
stuck in a motel, sharing the room with Fred and
Ethel.
Every two minutes, the train that passed right outside
the window would make the two beds vibrate so much
that they'd each move in different directions across
the room.
Priceless.

And every once in a while Lucy would display a
sardonic intelligence that we all saw as much closer to
the real Lucille Ball.
And that was great too.

When we started "Laverne & Shirley", we knew we
had physical comediennes, and that we'd be compared
to Lucy.
So we consciously attempted to do what we thought
Lucy did best--have the girls be victims of
circumstance.
Say what you will about "Laverne & Shirley", there
was never any scheming.

So faced with this ungodly task in front of me, I
decided to take the highest road possible--to have
Suzanne be the kind of Lucy who was a victim of
circumstance.

Into the valley of death.
There I went.

I decided to take the highest road I could, and make
her a victim of circumstance.
I was also trying to determine what my goal was.
The price of succeeding here was that Suzanne would
want to do this every week.
I don't know if I could stomach that.
Maybe it would work once.
As an aberration. As a fluke.

But doing it every week would rob the show of any shred of integrity it might have.
Maybe I was completely deluding myself.
Maybe the mere casting of Suzanne Somers cost the show any integrity it could ever hope to have.

I had had visions of what this show could be when I first got involved in it.

My show-runner hero of all time is Nat Hiken.
He was the man who created and ran "Sergeant Bilko". My favorite sitcom of all time.
He also created and ran "Car 54, Where Are You?"
One of my favorite sitcoms of all time.

I envisioned "She's The Sheriff" as being the sister-ship of "Car 54, Where Are You?"
It would be written in Nat Hiken style.
It's a very intelligent style.

I basically had to educate my rather neophyte writing staff about how to write in that style.
Once I did, I think they and I pulled it off very successfully.
I think this because the three hundred people who showed up as the live audience every week responded exactly as I hoped and expected they would.
The writers and I were the only ones who knew that we were trying to emulate Nat Hiken.
Us, and a few of my friends.

The Lorimar brass........perhaps brass is giving them too much credit.
The Lorimar tin always seemed rather surprised at how enthusiastic the audiences were every week.
I wasn't.

After shooting five episodes and never missing with the live audience, we were going to go on the air the following Tuesday.

The writers were getting excited.
They were saying things like "We can't miss with this show! The critics are going to love it!"

I said "Fellas, I don't want to burst your bubble here, but we're going to be lucky if we get one good review here."
They looked wounded.
I continued,
"What self-respecting Television critic is going to write 'You know, I watched this sitcom last night, She's The Sheriff, with Suzanne Somers with her bleached blonde hair and her long fingernails, being poured into a Sheriff's outfit, and it ranks right up there with the greats.
Mary Tyler Moore, move over!'
It's not going to happen. It doesn't matter how well written it is.
We are victims of packaging. It's like we're wearing a sign on our backs for the critics saying
Kick Me Hard".
And unfortunately, I have never been so right in my life.

The nicest thing written about this show was "You know, it wasn't nearly as bad as I thought it was going to be."
I turned that one into a plaque and hung it up in my office.
It was all I could cling to.

Years later, TV Guide listed the 50 Worst Sitcoms of All Time.
"She's The Sheriff" came in at number 45.
I'm pretty sure that the people who compiled the list had never even seen it.
I actually had three shows that made that list.
That tied me with Garry Marshall.
Nobody else had that many.
What are you going to do?

I had to ignore the reviews. I needed a reason to get up in the morning with enthusiasm.
So I just kept thinking that Nat Hiken would be looking down on me and smile.

I also had heard third-hand that Carl Reiner had watched the show and liked it a lot.
That helped.

If we failed at her being Lucy, maybe the problem would go away.
But again, at what cost?
Failing, with me, goes against the grain.
At bottom, I am a professional.
The goal is always to succeed.
I was going to try to succeed as best as I could, and deal with the next battle as it came up.

The best idea that any of us could come up with for a story under these circumstances dealt with an FBI agent who had always been a desk man.
This was his first assignment in the field.
He was also somewhat of a prankster, and on pure whim, figured out ways for the Sheriff and her deputies to essentially jump through hoops that he had created in order to make them look foolish, under the guise of a Sting Operation.
Doesn't look like much on paper, does it.
It didn't look like much on about forty-five pieces of paper either.
But I thought it had a prayer.
That was about it.
A prayer.

We did a table reading of it as the show we would do the following week.
Generally, after each reading, everyone would have their input.

Suzanne, knowing that this was our sop to her ambitions, championed the script.
The Lorimar tin were strangely non-committal.

They usually had far harsher notes about far better scripts.
Here, nothing.
They were going to let Suzanne and I twist in the wind on this one.

We had to cast the key part of the FBI agent.
Casting at Lorimar was always a sticky process.
Everything involved politics.
The head of casting, the late Barbara Miller, ruled the roost there.
She had her select favorites who kept showing up to audition for me, and I kept not casting them, because they weren't very good.
But they were on Barbara Miller's dance card, so they kept showing up, for me to reject.

So when actors showed up to read for the FBI agent, I once again got to see, as MAD Magazine used to put it, "The Usual Gang of Idiots".
As I was already in a compromising mood, and starting to piss off Barbara Miller by constantly rejecting her dance partners, I cast one of them.
He was less than wonderful.
He was less than good.
But that week, I was a beaten man, and figured that some fights are worth making, and this wasn't one of them.
So I was resigned to this pact I was making with the devil.

The Tuesday of the week of shooting, the actor we hired, whom I hadn't wanted in the first place, got sick and didn't show up.
He had to quit.

We had to replace him.
If this wasn't an omen, nothing was.

I was trying to turn Suzanne Somers into Lucille Ball.
A Rumplestilskinian task.

And the key guest actor, who I didn't want in the first
place, who was basically forced down my throat
politically, got sick and quit on Tuesday.
We were shooting on Friday.

I decided not to go down without a fight.
I was at least going to give it the old college try and
replace this actor with someone I thought was really
good.
Having gone to an old college, I did something I
hadn't done previously on this show.
I got out the Academy Players Directory, a large
dictionary-sized book that contained the names and
pictures of essentially the entire Los Angeles talent
pool.
The directory comes in a set of four books:
Leading Men, Leading Women, Male Characters and
Comedians, and Female Characters and
Comediennes.
I started looking through the Male Characters and
Comedians book.

A word to all aspiring actors:
If you are planning to change your name for
professional purposes, have your last name begin with
a letter towards the beginning of the alphabet.

These books are laid out alphabetically, and I and
everyone I know who has used these books start at the
beginning with "A", and proceed sequentially.
If you're in the back of the book, we'll never get to you.

So I was going to cast this one out of my head, finding someone whose work I liked and someone who I had worked with, who I could count on to at least put the best face on this show as possible in a key role.

The brilliant author, William Goldman, in his 1968 book, ""The Season", an essay-filled book about each play that opened on Broadway the previous year, discussed the musical "Golden Rainbow".
It starred Steve Lawrence and Eydie Gorme.
I saw it. I thought it was pretty bad.
Goldman saw it. He thought it was pretty bad.
Goldman noted how it went through many changes on its way to town and how a lot of people's brains were picked on how to improve it.
Goldman quoted someone. I forget who.
This person said, "It's exactly like washing garbage. No matter how much you wash it, when you get done, it's still garbage".

So when I opened the Characters and Comedians book to "A", I was determined to have garbage that was washed, cleaned, dry-cleaned, hand-pressed, and Martinized.
Nobody was going to say I didn't try to make it good.

I made it all the way up to the "G"s, and then I found him: Dick Gautier.

Remember Dick Gautier?
The original Conrad Birdie on Broadway in "Bye Bye Birdie"?
Hymie the Robot on "Get Smart"?
Robin Hood on "When Things Were Rotten"?

Too young to remember these?
So were the casting people foisted on me by Barbara Miller.

That's why they never thought to bring in anyone like Dick Gautier.

I'd worked with Dick Gautier on "Happy Days". He was brilliant.

I turned to one of the other producers, stared him down, and said "Get me Dick Gautier". Noticing the crazed look in my eyes, and not wanting to cross me, he executed my command.

Next morning, there was Dick Gautier, already rehearsing with the cast.

And he was actually bringing these scenes to life.

They finished the scene, and I went up to him and thanked him for being so terrific, and for jumping in like this at what was virtually the last minute, and I told him what a big fan of his I was. He looked at me and said "Then why did you wait so long to bring me in?"

To some questions, there are just no easy answers.

In Billy Wilder's great 1944 movie, "Double Indemnity", Edward G. Robinson played an unforgettable character named Barton Keyes. Barton Keyes was an insurance investigator. He was THE insurance investigator. If you wanted a claim investigated in 1944, Barton Keyes was who you wanted. As he told anyone who asked, he had "A little man inside him", who could sniff out a phony claim every time. "Nyaaahhh, see??!! Every Time!!!!

I've always felt that I had a "little man" inside of me, who could sniff out a problem with a script every time. Nyaahh see? Every time. He's never missed.

That's why, on most show nights, when about to face the three hundred people who comprised the live audience, I'd walk down to the stage, rubbing my hands together, thinking, "Boy, I can't wait until they see this!"

Because the "little man" inside me told me that I had successfully sniffed out any potential problem with the script.

If there was any screwing up to do, it would be by the actors. Not me.

During rehearsals, Dick Gautier was a riot.
He was cracking everybody up, especially me.
Even Barbara Miller conceded to me that he was a good idea.

On camera-blocking day, he killed the crew.
Suzanne, while no Lucy, was really funny.
The writers thought we'd actually pulled this one out.

But the "little man" inside of me was telling me otherwise.
The "little man" was saying that this episode was inherently stupid.
That the three hundred people would notice this, and this show would just lay there.

After the Thursday run-through, I gave minimal notes.
I didn't see the point of giving more than that.
The Lorimar execs had no notes.
For me or the actors.
Unprecedented.
All the actors were performing the hell out of it.
They could not be improved upon.

But we were still washing garbage.
I had never seen garbage washed so well.

So Friday night, I went down to the stage knowing
that we were going to fail.
The only things I wasn't certain of was to what degree
we were going to fail, and what the ramifications
would be.

The audience was in their usual great mood at the
beginning of the night, helped along by our
outstanding warm-up man.
And I kept thinking "It's only a matter of time before
they turn on us."

Now, you must understand how rare this situation
was for me.
I mostly experienced nothing but pre-anticipated
success.

And you must understand how common this situation
was for most studio and network executives.
They'd all experienced tons of shows tanking in front
of the live audiences.

They were all totally surprised that through seven
episodes, I was batting a thousand.
They'd never experienced this before.
But instead of expressing any kind of gratitude, they
had come to expect it by show number eight.

Again, the actors performed the hell out of it.
Dick Gautier was great.
And the show only got intermittent laughs.
I think I'm being charitable.

"Intermittent" is certainly less than satisfactory to me.
Especially for a show designed to crown Suzanne the
Reigning Queen of Comedy.
It had to be twice as funny as any other episode we
did, because it had no better than half the reality-base.

So what you saw was actors working twice as hard, and getting half the laughs.
Kind of like Shecky Greene's act.

I felt sorry for all concerned, and took absolutely no pride in being right.

The Lorimar execs were totally confused.
"We'd always gotten our laughs. What happened?"

This question allowed me my one mocking moment.
I told them "Fellas, you just didn't give me enough notes."

We had an after-show party every week.
This was the shortest one on record.

On the set the next week, we did a very brief post mortem.
Suzanne said to me "Was it my fault? Did I louse it up?"
I said "Suzanne, you played it as well as anyone could."
"Then what was the problem?", she asked.
"It was simply a bad idea", I said, without saying "I told you so".

To her credit, she never requested that she be Lucy ever again, and went back to completely trusting me.

The following week, her husband, Alan, never taking an opportunity to keep his mouth shut, said to me, during the very successful taping, that the audiences at this show just don't respond to Suzanne like they do in her show in Las Vegas.
To which I said, "And for that, Alan, you and Suzanne should be eternally grateful."

*****

Why I Told Suzanne Somers That "Three's Company" Was Shit, Part 1.

Why?

Well, for one, I was able to.
I had access and proximity to her, being the Executive Producer of a show she starred in.

For another, I have and had a stupid mouth.

And last, and certainly not least, "Three's Company" was, in fact, and indeed, shit.

I'll explain the last first.

Along the way, including the formation of "She's The Sheriff, I have had many dealings with the women involved with "Three's Company".
Joyce DeWitt, Priscilla Barnes, and then Suzanne.
For a while, the girl who played Chrissie in the second of three pilots for that series was my girlfriend.
So even though I rarely watched it, I knew its history quite well.

"Three's Company", in my mind, was a show that never deserved to live.

I think it was a show that was written by morons, for morons, and about morons.

Allow me to explain: I thought it had one good thing going for it---John Ritter.
He was an expert light comedian.
But the execution of the premise was insulting to any audience.

They were attempting to do French farce, ostensibly in the tradition of Moliere and Feydeau.

A character jumps to the wrong conclusion about
another or other characters, and based on that,
hilarity ensues.
Moliere and Feydeau understood that this was a very
valid premise for a play.

What the slobs who ran "Three's Company overlooked
is that it's not any kind of decent premise for a TV
series.

I watched the first four or five weeks of it, mainly
because of Ritter, and because I could not believe
what I was witnessing.
Every week, a supposedly intelligent character,
usually Joyce DeWitt, jumped to the wrong conclusion
about one or both of the other two.
Every week.
If she's not a moron, wouldn't she, by say the fourth
week, say to herself "Well, here I am, jumping to
another conclusion about something.
I was wrong the last three times.
Might it just be possible that I'm wrong this time?"
The thought never entered her head.
This made someone the audience was to perceive as
intelligent a moron.
By morons. About morons. For morons.
This translates to = Shit.

The week "Laverne and Shirley" went on the air and
became #1 in the ratings, Garry Marshall,
Lowell Ganz, and I were invited to Fred Silverman's
office at ABC, for the one and only time.
It was simply a glad-handing meeting.
A "Well done, fellows" meeting.
During this meeting, Silverman asked us to watch a
videotape of something ABC was developing.
He got on the phone and said "Hey Mike, bring in the
"Three's Company" tape.
We're going to run it."

Mike was Silverman's number two in command.
He tries to load the cassette into the VCR, which was
one of those bigger ones that preceded even Betamax.
I had one of these machines.
Mike spends literally about twenty minutes
unsuccessfully trying to load the cassette into the
VCR. He was baffled.
It seemed to be beyond him.
I'm thinking. "Look at this poor schmuck. Look at this
show he's putting on for us. He'll never get anywhere
in this business".
He finally loads the tape, and we watch the first pilot
of Three's Company".
Silverman asks for our opinions. I thought it was shit.
But even I had enough tact to tell him how wonderful
it was.
Silverman says, "But the casting's all wrong, isn't it?
Except for the guy."
Who were we to disagree?
But to me casting wasn't the problem.
My problem was "How do you sustain it?"
But I kept my thoughts to myself.
Okay, so I think I've made the case for "Three's
Company" being shit.
In Part 2, I'll explain why I relayed this piece of
information to Suzanne Somers.

Oh, and Mike? The schmuck who couldn't load the
tape? Who, in my eyes had no future in the business?
Michael Eisner.

So what the hell do I know?

*****

Why I Told Suzanne Somers That "Three's Company" Was Shit, Part 2.

Let me just start by saying that working with Suzanne Somers was primarily one of the most pleasant experiences I've ever had in the business.

She was and is charming, funny, down to earth, professional, and always striving to do the work as well as possible.

And as I said, I had totally gained her trust.

She had heard the 300 people that made up the live audience laughing uproariously every week, and thus figured I was doing something right.

Creatively, she completely placed herself in my hands, and never regretted it.

But she had this one minor peccadillo: She was averse to any changes in the script.

She worried that it would cause her to have trouble remembering her lines.

Now, you've got to understand that I come from the Garry Marshall school of "We keep re-writing until it's as good as we can make it in the time allotted to us".

This meant continually re-writing until the cameras started rolling on show-night.

My best work was usually on show day, the last day of rehearsal.

I always worked best with a gun to my head, flying by the seat of my pants, making last-minute little fixes.

Suzanne hated this most of all.

Jack Klugman and Tony Randall devoured material.

They kept wanting More and New, even if it wasn't necessary.

I can't tell you how many times Lowell and I were sent up to our office during the filming to write a new tag for that night's episode for Jack and Tony.

It was the same way on "Happy Days" and "Laverne and Shirley".

Not the tag part, but the willingness by the cast to have new material thrown at them.

Even during the filming.

Suzanne was not built that way.

She was too worried that she'd look foolish in front of the audience by forgetting her lines.

I told her "Are you kidding? They'll love you for it. I mean they don't exactly think you're a rocket scientist to begin with. This only enhances your image with them."

She was less than convinced.

I said "What's more important, that you know all your lines in front of 300 people, or that you forget lines here and there that we can cut out, but the show is twenty times better when we show it to millions of people?

She said "I don't know, when we were doing "Three's Company", we got our scripts two weeks in advance, and we never changed a word."

And I said "Yeah, but "Three's Company was shit!!!

You see, I didn't go out of my way to say "Three's Company was shit.
It just evolved naturally out of the discussion.

Trouper that she was, she adapted to my way of working.
And if she was insulted, she hid it well.

I was very proud of that show, and her work in it.

And I got to express myself.

*****

Your More Than Basic Hall Of Famer.

(Written on September 9, 2009)

The news reached everyone late last week that Hall of
Fame baseball broadcaster Ernie Harwell has an
inoperable cancerous tumor.
This may not mean as much to people who don't live
in the Detroit area, as I do.
Because in Detroit, Ernie Harwell walks on water.
There is no single individual who is as beloved in the
Detroit area as Ernie Harwell.
People here are devastated by this news.
Ernie Harwell is 91 years old. This sort of news
shouldn't be all that devastating.
It probably isn't all that devastating to him.
But the fixture he has been in Detroit has caused
many if not most to be inconsolable.

I didn't grow up in Detroit, listening to Ernie Harwell.
I grew up in New York, where my baseball
broadcasting heroes were Mel Allen, Red Barber, and
Vin Scully.
Ernie did some broadcasting in New York for the
Dodgers, but this was when I was too young to be
aware of it.
But I spent most of the 90's and this past decade in
Detroit, so I got my fair share of Ernie, and I got what
all the shouting was about.
Vin Scully has usually been touted as baseball's poet.
And he certainly has been.
But Ernie has been every inch the poet as Vin Scully.
On TV, like Scully, he knows when to talk, and when
not to.

On radio, he knows the importance of telling you what happened in the play, i.e. "was he safe or out?" before describing the play.

Unlike the slobs who are currently doing the radio broadcasts for the Tigers.
They'll tell you everything about the play before they tell you the result.

In the early 90's, the Tigers' owner decided to terminate Ernie's contract on demographic grounds.
You never heard such a brouhaha.
Next year, he was the ex-owner, and Ernie was back.

My path crossed with Ernie's last year.
It turns out he lives about six blocks away from me, in a lavish retirement community.

The people who run the facility were always looking to provide live entertainment for their sumptuous 300 seat theatre.
Somebody knew somebody, and it led to interest on their part for them to have one of my plays performed there.

Ernie was on the Entertainment Committee.
This essentially made the difference between my caring and not caring about doing it.
So I did a reading of the play for the Entertainment Committee, got to meet Ernie, and got his approval.

That meant more to me than most things.
And we got to talk baseball.
Just me and Ernie. Shootin' the breeze.
He was delightful. A complete gentleman.

I put a production of the play on for their audience, and it played like gangbusters.

Ernie, quite pleased, congratulated me, and I felt like a trillion dollars.

He is one of those people who makes this planet better by his presence.

One more thing about that production---the leading male character is a sportscaster.

There's a line early on where he's trying to convince his mother that he's not famous.
To illustrate, he introduces himself to a cocktail waitress as Joe Garagiola.
The waitress buys into it.
This always gets a big laugh.
With Ernie's permission, we changed Joe Garagiola to Ernie Harwell.

Screams like you've never heard.

*****

124

A Beautiful Day For A Ballgame.

From Ernie Harwell,
Thursday, May 6th, 2010:

Yes fans, it's an absolutely beautiful day out here at
Comerica Park, and there are a whole lot of fans here
to be part of it.
I wish I was around to see it.
Well, maybe I am.
It depends on what you believe.
The Detroit Tigers are playing the Cleveland Indians
in the opening of a three game series.
But not here.
And not until tomorrow.
In Cleveland.
The fans here today are here to see me.
I'm lying in state, right here at the main entrance, and
I'll be here all day and night, until the last fan leaves.
I didn't want any public memorials.
The Tigers' owners have honored my wishes, and
months ago, we agreed on this public viewing, and I'm
honored to receive it.
I insisted that there would be free parking for all who
came, and that cold water and hot coffee be offered to
those in line.
The lines are very very long.
Thousands and thousands of people.

You know, I should have specified what kind of piped-
in music would be played.
This stuff is quite maudlin, serious, and depressing.
A bit dirge-like.
I think I would have preferred "Take Me Out To The
Ballgame".
Even if it was played in this tempo.

In the middle of the line, I see Mark Rothman.
I really didn't expect to see him.
He almost never leaves the house.
And he hates standing in lines.
He must have really liked me.

I met and spoke with him several times.
He told me how he grew up in New York, and how Vin
Scully was his God of sportscasting.
And how he spent about ten years in Detroit listening
to me, and that I was at least as good.
I think he meant it as a complement.
At least that's how I took it.
But then, I seem to be known for my graciousness.

There sure are a lot of youngsters here.
Each with their mothers , or fathers, or both.
These kids certainly never heard me call a game.
They're too young.
They probably have no idea why they're here.
I can hear fathers telling their children "Just be glad
you're here. Eventually, it will be a moment you'll
never forget."
That's certainly nice to hear.

Rothman is getting closer. He just accepted a cup of
cold water from one of the attendants.
He's wearing a Tigers cap.
It looks pretty good on him.
He's also wearing a Tigers T-Shirt.
It's hanging very loose on him.
That makes sense.
Since the last time I saw him, he's lost a lot of weight.
He looks very good.
He has the kind of physique that would look
particularly good in a Tigers home uniform.

We could sure use his bat in the lineup.
Too bad he can't field.
He's good-hit, no glove.
I guess he can always be a DH.
Except that he's so slow.
If he hit a home run, it would take him a month to get around the bases.

Here he comes.....right near the casket.
He's holding up the cup of water.
He's toasting me with it.
A tear is falling from his left eye.
Figures.
He's a lefty.
Bats left, throws left.....cries left.
He's waving good-bye to me.
Good-bye, Mark.

From Rothman:

Good-bye Ernie.
It was an honor to have met you, talked to you, and be at Comerica to see you last Thursday.
It has been a great reason to be in Detroit.

*****

Why I Get Creeped Out Watching "The Little Rascals"

Well, let's see.

There's the fact that one of them became a murderer (R.Blake), that one of them was shot to death in a barroom brawl, (Alfalfa), that the production values were the worst, much like anything that came out of the Hal Roach Studios:

Incredibly grainy shadowy film stock, the constant re-use of what we would call diddly music, which they shared with Laurel and Hardy.

The depiction of fathers (particularly Darla's father) as the wimpiest of men........

I'm sure they paid those kids in the dark.

But these are the kinds of things that could creep ANYBODY out.

What has creeped ME out in particular were a couple of personal encounters with a couple of former Rascals.

First: It's 1965.

I'm working as a page at ABC in New York.

ABC has a late night show called "Nightlife" that they are throwing to the wolves against Johnny Carson.

It was hosted by the now late Les Crane.

My duties as a page on that particular day was to be handed a list of that night's guests, and escort them to their dressing rooms.

I go to the set, and am handed the list.

I look it over.

I see the name "Darla Hood".

Rarely using my mouth as a tongue depressor, I say, out loud, "Darla Hood? Where'd they dig HER up from?"

Standing right next to me, a short, attractive 45 year-old woman stared daggers up at me and said "I'M Darla Hood!"

She didn't see the humor.
I felt terrible.
I'm amazed I wasn't fired.
I probably would have been if she had been
considered important enough.

Cut to 1977: I'm exec producing a series called
"Busting Loose".
There was a black character in it, and we decided to
do a show about his family. Showing up at the
auditions was the actor who played "Stymie" in the
Little Rascals.
Looking just like Stymie did as a kid, except he was
about 58.
I thought this was too good an opportunity to pass up.
So I cast him.
He was great in the show.
The live audience recognized him immediately and
gave him entrance applause.

About a week later, I get a call from Stymie.
He was bellyaching about how little he got paid for the
gig, and how he's having trouble making the rent, and
how somehow this was my fault.
And he started to put the touch on me.
He wanted me to lend him money.
Money I just knew I would never get back.
He was already known for his drug addictions.
I politely declined.
He hung up on me. So just about the only "Little
Rascals" I can watch are the ones where Jackie Cooper
had a hard-on for Miss Crabtree.
This was pre-Darla.
But if Stymie showed up in them, which he did
occasionally, I'd have to quickly shut it off.

*****

Another Show Business Relic.

At just about the time I unfortunately met Darla
Hood, who certainly could accurately then be
described as a show business relic, I also stumbled
upon another show business relic.
This one of the inanimate variety.

At virtually the same location.

Beneath the studio where "ABC Nightlife was taped,
was the pages locker room.

A seemingly quite ordinary locker room.
But I believe that it contained a secret.

A piece of show business history that probably
belonged in a museum.
But it wasn't in a museum.

It was right there, in the basement, in the ABC pages
locker room.
Unnoticed by anyone else.

I never called to anyone else's attention.
I think that was because I wanted it to be my own
personal secret.
I also think that either nobody else would care, or that
nobody else would believe me.

I'm revealing this for the first time.
Maybe you won't care or believe me either.
I'll take my chances:

It was the locker next to mine.
All the lockers were a drab olive green.
On the locker door next to mine, in very faint black
letters, it said:
"Lt. J.G. D.A. Roberts."

Maybe this means nothing to you.
What it meant to me was "Mister Roberts".

That this was most-likely the locker used on the set of
the Broadway production of "Mister Roberts", some
eighteen years previously.
I couldn't and can't think of any other logical
explanation.

When Broadway shows close, their sets are usually
carted off somewhere in the metropolitan area to die,
or be destroyed.
It's more than possible that around 1950, when "Mr.
Roberts" closed in New York, and ABC was beginning
its fledgling TV broadcasting, somebody realized that
they were going to need pages.
And the pages would need a locker room.
And lockers.
And that somebody had seen "Mr. Roberts", knew it
was closing, and asked if he could have the lockers
from "Mr. Roberts" for the ABC pages locker room.
And this somebody was probably told "Sure. All you
have to do is show up with a truck and haul them
away".

It's more than more than possible.
It is more than more than likely.
There had been no other productions of "Mister
Roberts in the metropolitan area in the intervening
years.
This must be the explanation.

So I am convinced that for about two years, I was
dressing and undressing right next to history.
How many other people do you know who can say
that, and mean it?

******

Gene Barry.

I met Gene Barry on April 18th, 1987.
It's a date that stands out to me as much as November 22nd, 1963, and September 11th, 2001.

Not necessarily because it was the day I met Gene Barry, although that was certainly a significant factor.

And I didn't have any anticipation that I would be meeting Gene Barry that day.
It wasn't "Oh, goody, goody goody! Today I get to meet Gene Barry!

I didn't know that he was going to be where I was.

It was where I was that was primarily the significant part.

Harry Crane was a great comedy writer.

After working with him on "Happy Days", I decided to hire him as one of the writers on "She's The Sheriff", mainly so he could impart his wisdom on our very young staff, and provide me someone to have lunch with every day.

Harry was approaching 75. And, I guess he felt it appropriate to invite me to his birthday party at his home in Beverly Hills.
I, of course, was delighted to attend.

I had no idea how delighted until I got there.

The other guests were comprised of just about everyone I'd ever seen and/or idolized on TV since I was a little kid:

Within two rooms, where I was allowed to mingle freely, were, among others, Sid Caesar, Danny Thomas, Phyllis Diller, Jan Murray, Steve Allen, Jack Carter, Audrey Meadows.......and Gene Barry.

This turnout was a major indication of how much Harry was loved by the major league show business community of his time.
And I was introduced to all as his "boss", which provided me with instant acceptance.

I overheard Jan Murray tell this gut wrenching story about how he lost his brother in the fighting in World War II. Someone was reading the casualty list and told Jan that he had nothing to worry about. No Murray's here. Just some guy named Janofsky.
Janofsky was Jan's real last name.
So in trying to be comforting, this guy inadvertently told Jan that he had lost his brother.

Danny Thomas was bemoaning the fact that there was no place for storytellers in nightclubs any more.

I told Audrey Meadows how much I loved her as Alice Kramden, and she immediately hit me up for work.
At that moment, I only wished that I had some work to provide for her.

This was all like strolling down the halls of the Museum of Broadcasting.

I'm just giving you a taste of the trappings, the event.

To me, a major, major, unforgettable event.

The main topic of discussion at Harry Crane's birthday party on April 18th, 1987 was the death, the previous night, of comedian Dick Shawn, who actually died in the middle of a performance of his one-man show, onstage, while all the audience members thought it was part of the act.

Dick Shawn was one of the most inventive, imaginative, daring comedians we've ever had.

Without Dick Shawn, I doubt that there ever would have been an Andy Kaufman.

Dick Shawn was truly a high wire act. He was the original Great Wallendas of comedy.
And like many of the Wallendas, he came to a similar end.

From his IMDB Biography:

"The irony of his death on stage is that it went "unnoticed" because of Shawn's strict instructions to stage crews. He would tell all concerned that he was liable to do anything at any time, including pratfalls, and that they were not to react to this. At his last performance, it did not occur to anyone that something tragic had happened until it was felt that his lying motionless on stage had run the joke rather thin. It was only then that Shawn was discovered to have died doing what he did best; enthralling his audience with his marvelous humor."

Dick Shawn was a major influence on me.

When I was 16, graduating High School, I decided I didn't want to go to the Prom.
Instead, I took this lovely young girl with me to see Dick Shawn in the original production of
"A Funny Thing Happened on the Way to the Forum".
He had replaced Zero Mostel, and was absolutely brilliant.
To this day, I have never seen anyone own a stage the way he did that night.

And I thought and said to myself: "Him. That's what I want to be, is Him."

When I went to college, and started getting cast in plays there, it was all with the idea of becoming, somehow, some way, Him.

Two years later, the Theatre Department at Queens College was putting on a production of "Forum". My opportunity to be Him was at hand. But I was thwarted by the director, one of the students, who didn't see it that way. He offered me one of the other parts. I wasn't going to be Him. It was a good part, so I took it. But I still wasn't going to be Him.

The director and I went at it like cats and dogs. I thought he was a prick. He thought I was a shmuck. We were probably both right.

He would pontificate at the drop of a beret about how Directing was his chosen profession. He was nineteen, for chrissakes, but he had chosen his profession. And I would say something a propos, like "Choose this!" in front of everybody. Probably a main reason why I wasn't invited to the cast party.

When I was doing "She's The Sheriff", 20 years later, the editor told me that she knew the guy who had chosen his profession. She played tennis with him. I said "Tell him I play tennis. I'd love to play with him some time." This offer went unheeded. Most-likely because in the ensuing years, Directing had not chosen him. His biggest credit had been in the 70s, when he was an Associate Producer on a syndicated show called "Lie Detector", which starred F. Lee Bailey. This was one of my favorite shows, by the way.

I'll write about it some day.
If you look at Chosen Profession's credits in the most
recent edition of the Writers Guild Directory, his job
on "Lie Detector" still looms largest, with very little
else following.
Why I believe in God.

So I never got to be Dick Shawn, but at least I'm here
to tell about it.

Later that evening, I turned my attention to fawning
out loud over Sid Caesar, telling him that he was to
television what the Marx Brothers were to movie fans
of my generation. He seemed very flattered.
This was all within earshot of Jack Carter and Danny
Thomas, but I didn't give a shit.
After all, I was the same guy who told Chosen
Profession to "Choose This!" in front of everybody.

Then I noticed Gene Barry.
He hadn't opened his mouth all evening. He just
seemed to be drinking in everything everyone was
saying.
And I realized that I had something I wanted to tell
him.
Something that meant a lot to me.

I have, upon occasion, alluded to my mother.
To elaborate about her a little bit, the woman was
always capable, and used her capabilities quite often,
to embarrass me in public and in private.
And she provided the capability for me to return the
gesture in kind.
In short, we would consistently drive each other crazy.
We would go the full fifteen rounds with each other.
(In those days, championship fights would go fifteen
rounds. Now it's only twelve. Pity.)

BUT, and this is a major BUT, which is why I've capitalized it twice, there was probably nobody who was ever more protective of anyone's well-being as she was of mine.
Probably much to my father's dismay.
This woman adored me.
I'm certain that she adored me more than I deserved being adored.
I'm sure more than my father thought I deserved being adored.

She died in 1983, at the age of 61, after spending fifteen years with all sorts of agonizing cancer.

I didn't cry at the funeral. I had gotten it all out as she was on her deathbed the day she died.

My two aunts looked at me askance for my not showing any emotion at the funeral.
I questioned my own detachment about it for weeks afterwards.

About three months later, I went to see the hugely successful musical "La Cage Aux Folles" on Broadway.
It is a GREAT show.
Gene Barry and George Hearn starred in it, as a gay couple who have raised a son.
Barry ran a nightclub in St. Tropez, and Hearn was its star, the drag queen, Zaza.
Gene Barry had only been one of those guys who had had a couple of successful TV series,
"Bat Masterson" and "Burke's Law".
I wasn't expecting all that much from him or the show.
But I did and do love Jerry Herman's music and lyrics every time out, and he always writes upbeat, and the source material was very funny, so I expected to have a grand old time.
And I was having that grand old time, until Gene Barry sang a song that completely devastated me.

Because I was thinking about my mother when he
sang it.
It wiped me out when I saw it.
I was literally crying like a baby.
It still wipes me out just thinking about it and writing
about it.

It occurs because George Hearn's son won't invite him
to his wedding because of his gay lifestyle, afraid he'd
show up in drag. Gene Barry magnificently sings this
song to the son, basically to shame him into changing
his mind, with George Hearn, in drag, looking on:

I don't know if you have ever heard it, but here at
least, are the lyrics (he said, through tears):

"How often is someone concerned with the tiniest
thread of your life?
Concerned with whatever you feel and whatever you
touch?

Look over there.
Look over there.
Somebody cares that much.

How often does somebody sense that you need them
without being told?
When you have a hurt in your heart you're too proud
to disclose?

Look over there.
Look over there.
Somebody always knows.

When your world spins too fast,
And your bubble has burst,
Someone puts himself last,
So that you can come first.

So count all the loves who will love you from now 'til the end of your life,

And when you have added the loves who have loved you before,

Look over there.
Look over there.

Somebody loves you more..."

They virtually had to carry me out of the theatre on a stretcher.

I told an abbreviated version of this story to Gene Barry.
He seemed touched, and pleased that I told him.

I guess the one I really wanted to tell this to, was Jerry Herman.
But he wasn't in the room.

This was the next best thing.

If you want to hear "Look Over There", as sung by Gene Barry on the "La Cage Aux Folles" cast album, e-mail me at macchus999@aol.com and I can forward you instructions as to how to easily get to it on the web, for free.

November 22nd, 1963
September 11th, 2001
and April 18th, 1987.

And not necessarily in that order.

*****

Actors Must Think.

I believe that Truman Capote was the first to point out the inverse correlation between one's intelligence and one's ability to be a good actor.
I believe he put it this way---"Have you ever met Marlon Brando? He's as dumb as they come."

He wasn't referring to book larnin'.
He was alluding to good ole common sense.

It has been my experience that Capote pretty much knew what he was talking about.

I'm a pretty good actor, and it's certainly true in my case.
Except for acting and writing, I am a complete nitwit.

But at least I think while I am acting or writing.

I have witnessed examples of good actors who suddenly stop thinking in the line of duty.

I'll describe a couple of instances.
Both of them involve episodes of "The Odd Couple".

We did an episode with Alex Karras (no, this isn't about you, Alex, if you're out there) where he played a pro football player Oscar interviews, and Felix meets his wife and inadvertently falls in love with her.
It was a pretty good episode.
So good, that when I was doing "New Odd CUPPle", we did it again.
There was another actor in the original episode.
I'm not going to mention his name here.
He passed away several years ago, and I needn't besmirch him by name.

I'll drop a couple of hints, though.

He was in the original cast of one of the most
acclaimed musicals of all time, and was part of a trio
that sang one of the most acclaimed musical opening
numbers of all time in it.
The really ambitious among you don't even need these
hints.
He was a very reliable, pretty talented character actor.
In this episode, he played Alex Karras's football coach
in the locker room.

In life, this actor had a particular affectation.
He wore a beret all the time.
This certainly belied the kind of characters he was
usually cast as.
Maybe he was trying to avoid getting typed.
The fact that he had a Brooklyn accent didn't help his
cause.

He didn't appear in the episode until the next to last
scene.

I didn't get to see them shoot that scene, or the last
one.
Because I was doing what I was sometimes recruited
to do:
Going back to my office and writing a new tag.
The tag is the brief scene right after the last
commercial.

Jack and Tony were never happy with the tags we
provided.
They were in fact never happy with anything that had
a shelf life of more than an hour.

So the only part of the rest of the show that I had seen
filmed was the tag we had just written.

I was told that the rest of the show had gone really
well.

I wasn't surprised. Alex Karras was wonderful in rehearsals.

Cut to: The screening of the first rough cut, about a week later.
I couldn't believe what I saw.
You're probably all way ahead of me by now, but for those of you with not all that much imagination, here goes:
There was the actor who played the football coach, STILL WEARING THE BERET!

You know. Like ALL football coaches do.

It never occurred to him that this might be out of character, inappropriate.

In all fairness to the actor, I was the only one who noticed.
The director, the producers, the other writers, they didn't notice when it was being filmed or at the screening.
When I pointed it out at the screening, everyone was embarrassed.
But not the actor. He wasn't there.

And this piece of ridiculousness will be seen as long as there are reruns and DVDs.

When we did the episode on "New Odd CUPPle", we got Ernie Hudson, and made him a fighter instead of a football player. He didn't have a coach.
He had a trainer.
And the trainer wasn't wearing no esteenkin' beret.

About fifteen years later, when I was doing "She's The Sheriff", the original actor in question would show up regularly at the Lorimar commissary to have lunch with himself and his beret.

To be seen, I guess.
Just seeing the beret gave me the hives.
My secretary and I were having lunch there one day
when he was there.
She knew him, and his work.
She said "He's such a sweet little man. Why don't you
hire him sometime?"

I turned to her, thought for a moment, and simply
said "Don't get me started."

Next:

We did an episode of "The Odd Couple" where it is
decided that Felix and Oscar should hire a
housekeeper.
Felix sees this as an opportunity for things to run
more smoothly when he's not around.
Oscar sees this as an opportunity to get laid.
That was the conflict.
On that show, there was always a mandated conflict.
That was the conflict for that week.

Among the interviewees for this position was a
"Jewish Mother" type, played by a very funny older
actress named Janet Brandt.
At the first run-through on Wednesday, she took what
was a modest amount of dialogue and completely
killed.

The writers, the producers, the director, Jack and
Tony. Killed.
At that night's rewrite session, Tony and Jack agreed
on what was for them a rare magnanimous gesture.
They wanted us to pad her part.
Did I say rare?
I think I meant unique.
Tony and Jack were extremely generous to one
another.
And no one else.

It used to drive Tony crazy when Al Molinaro got laughs with extremely little effort.
But an outsider? This sort of generosity was unheard of around these parts.

Janet knew she had scored in that first run-through. Seeing how much more she had in the script the next day only reinforced her opinion of herself.

Her son had appeared on another "Odd Couple" episode previously, and, if I'm not mistaken, received the usual outside actor treatment from Tony and Jack. The same way one would treat dirt.

Unless they weren't on speaking terms, you'd have to think that mother and son probably discussed this.

An intelligent actress armed with this knowledge, or even without this knowledge, would be very, very cautious, and approach this situation with as much restraint as possible.
In the Fonda family tradition.

Not Janet.
Remember. This was a very very good, very funny actress.
But at the Thursday night run-through, she milked her part dry.
She overacted, mugged, upstaged the stars, and thoroughly embarrassed herself and everyone watching.
And she thought she was killing again.

In a prizefight, if one of the boxers gets knocked down and appears groggy, the referee will often ask him, once he's risen to his feet, "What town are you in?" and "Who are you fighting?"

If the boxer gives the correct answers, he's usually allowed to continue.

Metaphorically, an actor must always know what town he or she is in, and who he or she is fighting.

Needless to say, at that night's rewrite session, the edict was not only to take away what was added to her part from Wednesday to Thursday, but to also cut down what she originally had on Wednesday, to virtually nothing.

Lee, the #1 Odd Couple fan on my website and probably the world, waxed ecstatically about how wonderful she was in that episode.

I told him "Lee, you should have seen her on Wednesday".

*****

Horton Hears A Hooray.

So a couple of weeks ago, I was channel surfing.
And I stumbled upon a movie on Turner Classic
Movies called "Little Miss Big Shot", from 1935.
It had just started five minutes previously.
I see Edward Everett Horton is in it.
I hit the record button on the Tivo immediately.
That's what I do whenever I see Edward Everett
Horton is in anything.
Except "F Troop".
I don't want to remember him as the ancient
Chief Roaring Chicken.
But that's me.
Unfortunately, that's how most people remember him.
It was not his best work.
It's impossible to do your best work on "F Troop".

Every once in a while, when Letterman has an actor or
actress on that he really wants to butter up, he'll tell
him or her that there isn't a movie made that wouldn't
be better if this person wasn't in it.
Well, before "F Troop", this was absolutely true of
Edward Everett Horton.

So a few days later, I watch "Little Miss Big Shot".
Missing the first five minutes didn't hurt anything.
It's Warner Brothers' blatant ripoff of "Little Miss
Marker", the Shirley Temple vehicle of the year
before.
Same plot.
It's title even began with "Little Miss".
Nobody ever had any shame.
It was designed to launch a little girl named
Sybil Jason to be their Shirley.
She was cute, but certainly no Shirley.

Robert Armstrong, of "King Kong" fame, had the
Adolphe Menjou part.
And Edward Everett Horton was his sidekick.

I love movies made in the 30's. All the men wore hats,
they all needed two hands to use the telephone, they
all began sentences with "Say...."
There was STYLE.

They gave Sybil Jason a dog. A really cute dog.
And the dog figured in the plot.
Being a 1935 Warner Brothers picture, there were
gangsters, and too much violence.
So they didn't quite capture "Little Miss Marker".
All it really had going for it was Edward Everett
Horton.
And it was enough.

Horton was in a lot of scenes with little Sybil and the
dog.
The old axiom for actors is "Never appear in scenes
with kids or dogs. You won't have a chance".

The axiom for kids and dogs should be "Never appear
in scenes with Edward Everett Horton.
You won't have a chance."

You simply can't take your eyes off of him.
And he's consistently hilarious.
As always.
Verbally and visually.
He invented the comic technique of starting to answer
a question he had no intention of answering, and then
catching himself in the process.
If he didn't invent it, he perfected it.
He is the master of the triple-take.
He's probably the best comic character actor we've
ever had.

In all those Astaire and Rogers pictures that he was in, great as the two of them were, I kept waiting for them to get off the dance floor so that the camera would again be on Horton, doing his best to move those stupid plots along.

A good actor-friend of mine named Jim Cox, who actually introduced me to my lovely wife, once lived in Horton's guest house, and they became good friends. I don't know how much of an influence Horton had on Jim, but Jim had many of Horton's mannerisms and acting traits. He was wonderful in one of my plays, and I saw Horton in him when I cast him.

Jim told me a story about how Horton would complain because the author of a play called "Springtime For Henry", which Horton would tour in for decades, tried to sue him because Horton essentially cut and rewrote much of the play, because it needed much cutting, rewriting, and improving.
Horton would say "That ingrate! I'm the only one who performs that rotten play of his!
If it wasn't for me, he wouldn't receive a nickel for it! I've singlehandedly made him a wealthy man, and that bastard is suing me!"
Hearing Jim tell this story, sounding exactly like Horton in the process, is worth any price of admission.

If you've got Tivo and Turner Classic Movies, I'd advise you to regularly do a search for movies that Horton is in.
Turner has most of 'em, and show 'em all the time.
It's a major opportunity to treat yourself.
You'll thank me.

*****

Firing An Actress You Didn't Want To Fire, Not Firing An Actress You Did Want To Fire, And Getting Fired By An Actress You Didn't Want To Fire You.

I'll start with the last one first.

This was more than twenty years ago. One of my plays was being done in Los Angeles.
The producer knew Donna Pescow.
You know, "Saturday Night Fever", "Angie", and out.
This was shortly after "Angie" and Donna Pescow was perceived as a name that would fill seats.
I'd seen "Angie", and, while not overwhelmed by her comedy chops, I thought overall that she would be an asset.
Larry Miller had already agreed to do the male lead.
Larry had and has enormous comedy chops.
At the time, he was way shy on acting chops.
He knew it, and eagerly placed himself in my hands.
To this day, he will credit me for turning him into an actor.

Donna Pescow read the play, and agreed to do the female lead.
Larry and I met with her at her high-rise apartment in Westwood.

They read out loud the first scene they had together.
I was not encouraged.
There were many things that were funny in that scene that weren't funny the way they came out of her mouth.
Trying not to seem too intrusive, I let them keep reading until the scene was mercifully over.

It was decision time.
Do I have to give her line readings to make this work?
Will she be receptive to line readings?
If she is, will it help?
If she isn't, can I live with what she's doing, and is
there any other way to convey my attitude about her
complete misinterpretation of the material?
You can talk all you want to her about character, but
what it all boils down to is that this character would
say a certain line a certain way.
If she doesn't see that, then she sees a different
character.
And not as good a character as the one I wrote.

It's moments like those that make me wonder why
she'd agree to do the play in the first place.
If that's the way she heard it, then what she was
hearing was a shitty play.
I would much rather not have to give line readings as
a director of a comedy.
But I'm greedy.
I want to elicit every single laugh that I know a script
contains.
And I constantly hope that I will be surprised by an
actor who finds a legitimate laugh that I didn't realize
was there.
These actors do exist.
Cindy Williams did it all the time.
As did Tony Randall.

This is my attitude about directors giving line
readings:
It depends on who's giving them and how much
respect you have for that person.

If I'm an actor, and the director's giving me bad line
readings, then I hate line readings.

If the director is giving me good line readings, line readings that are better than the way I'm reading them, then I embrace that director and love line readings.

I've been in both situations.

When Jack Lemmon and Walter Matthau did movies with Billy Wilder, Wilder constantly gave them line readings, and they both lapped them up.
Because they had the highest regard for Billy Wilder.
When they worked with the poor schmuck who directed "Grumpy Old Men", they wouldn't give him the time of day.
To them, that director was Rodney Dangerfield.

Neil Simon is famous for giving line readings to everyone.
But second hand, through the director.
So there are a lot of actors who probably hate Gene Saks.
I've had actors tell me that they don't want line readings because it deprives them of the fun of discovering the right way to do it for themselves.
I've often had to remind them that acting isn't necessarily supposed to be fun.
It's supposed to be WORK.
You're usually getting paid for it.
It's supposed to be fun for the AUDIENCE.
THEY'RE the ones who paid to get in.
Sometimes you don't have time for the actors to discover it for themselves.
And sometimes they NEVER discover it.
Fun for the actor is by necessity a luxury.

So to me, it was a no brainer.
I had to give Donna Pescow line readings.
We did the scene again, with me interrupting her and giving her line readings.
I commenced.
She bristled.

She seemed to have little regard for Larry, and seemed
to feel singled out because I didn't give HIM any line
readings.
What she didn't know is that I'd already gone over the
entire play with Larry, and he had already lapped up
my input.
I had the feeling that she thought she was slumming
anyway, and certainly had a misplaced lack of respect
for me.
She bailed after that one and only rehearsal.
So even though I was still there and she was gone, I
felt like I was fired by an actress.

Who's to say why careers turn sour?
In Donna Pescow's case, I'm guessing that she was
perceived as nothing special.
It's just possible that if she had placed herself in my
hands, we might have fooled enough people to think
otherwise.
Who knows? It might have made a difference.
Just a guess.

Next Case:

I guess I'm going in reverse order.

I don't like firing anyone.
I really don't.
I know some producers, who, when someone has to be
fired, raise their hand and say "May I do it?"
I'm not one of those type people.
I regard having to fire someone as a personal failure
on my part.
That I made the wrong choice to begin with.
I've fired very few people.
I once fired my secretary, and simultaneously
recommended her for a much better job as a Studio
Executive, which she got, based on my
recommendation.
So I like to think that I always mean well.

I did another production of the same play Donna
Pescow didn't do.
It was in Florida, seven years ago.
It ended up being very successful.
But it was a rocky Road to Morocco.
The actress who auditioned for the lead and was cast
was excellent.
For the most part, during rehearsals, she was
excellent.
Throughout the run, she was excellent, although she
often experienced brain farts that left her fellow actors
terrified.
For them, it was a little like riding down the rapids on
the African Queen.
But she scored with the audience consistently.

However, there was one run-through about three days
before we opened, where I wanted to fire her.
Let me amend that.
I wanted to kill her.
During that run-through, she was absolutely dreadful.
No sense of character.
No sense of comedy.
Both of which were amply on display in all the other
rehearsals.

Now anyone can be dreadful on any given night.
Particularly during a rehearsal.
But ordinarily, that's no reason for firing or killing.
It's a reason for being confused, which is what I was.

I had to address this with her after the run-through.
And I didn't want to embarrass her by doing it in
public.
So I said, "Robin, can I speak to you backstage?"
She huffily followed me backstage.
I started to ask her the equivalent of "Ma Nishtatah"--
-Yiddish for "Why is this night different from all other
nights?"

She cut me off and said "How can you embarrass me like this? Everybody now knows that you called me back here to chew me out"
This at least showed an awareness that she stunk out the joint.
This begged several questions:
Was I not supposed to say anything?
If I was, should I have said it in front of everyone else?
Should I have been more diplomatic?
She then said "I always have at least one rehearsal where I'm off my game. Why is that so hard to understand?"
I. of course was thinking, "It's so hard to understand because you NEVER TOLD ME THIS BEFORE!!!!" and "Hey!! I don't know the proper etiquette when somebody stinks out the joint!"
She was making quitting noises.
We didn't have an understudy.
We were both getting a decent piece of change to do this show, so I really didn't take the quitting noises seriously.
Robin left that night in a snit, and when she showed up the following evening, she returned with it.
I don't like hurting anyone's feelings, whether they have it coming or not.
So I then found myself in the uncomfortable-for-more-than-one-reason position of being on my knees apologizing to this person who wasn't worthy of pressing my pants, just on the basis of her actions the previous night.
Why?
The show must go on.
And I wanted the tension and my bellyache to go away.
We were going to spend the next entire month together, and I wanted it to be as painless as possible.
When you stink, it's your fault and nobody else's.

And it's your responsibility to apologize to the director and the cast for stinking.
Particularly when you know you stunk.

If I had a decent understudy in place I would have fired Robin's ass that night.
And hoped that there wasn't a gun at my disposal.

Last Case:

There's always a pecking order.

As I've indicated before, you start out wanting Olivier or Brando, and you usually end up with Elliot Gould or George Segal.
And everyone in-between is part of the pecking order.
I guess if your pecking, Segal just noses out Gould.

When I did my two-character play in L.A. about ten years ago, the idea was to have the lead actress role split time-wise between the name actress we used and a semi-name actress.
Mainly, because I couldn't get the name actress to commit full-time.
If I could, I would have just gone with her and an understudy.

This and other things led to both of them at separate times chewing me out big time over the phone.

One, the name actress, because I couldn't commit to her yet because I was dickering with a bigger name actress.
The semi-name actress, because she was word perfect on the script and the name actress wasn't and "isn't that worth something?" and "Why do you keep changing the schedule to accommodate her and do nothing to accommodate me?"
The reasons for all of this, is of course, pecking order.

We planned an opening weekend rather than an opening night so that both actresses could get their share of the reviews.
About two weeks before opening, the semi-name actress had a potential major health crisis that led to her almost dropping out and missing several rehearsals.
It was touch and go.
I needed a third actress.
Someone with a very good reputation with a following in local L.A. theatre gave a very good audition and volunteered to step into the breach.
We didn't know what was going to happen with the semi-name actress.
This third actress, let's call her Evelyn, mainly because I don't remember what her name was (It might actually have been Evelyn) had only one demand: that she be part of opening weekend and get reviewed.
Even if she didn't demand it, I would have offered it.

The semi-name actress recuperated, bristled somewhat at having a three-way share of opening weekend, but she knew that Evelyn was doing us all a "large".
Of course, Evelyn was also doing herself a "large".
Nobody's that selfless.
Evelyn had her first performance during preview week.
She was quite wonderful.
The semi-name actress went on the next night.
She was also quite wonderful, as I knew she would be, because I'd worked with her many times.
Evelyn went on the following night, and I had to fumigate the stage afterwards.
She had completely lost it, and was god-awful.
I gave notes on stage afterwards to both actors which essentially went "I don't know what went on up there tonight, but it certainly wasn't my play".

The difference between this and what happened with Robin in Florida is that Evelyn had no clue that she had stunk up the place.

The clock was ticking.
I knew what I had to do.
I didn't like having to do it.
I called Evelyn's husband, who was also an actor and served as her intermediary.
I told him that I'd have to remove Evelyn from the opening weekend rotation.
I'd be willing to give her an occasional performance once we had opened, but I couldn't risk what happened last night happening in front of reviewers.
This wasn't Florida.
This is L.A., where my reputation is on the line.
And I had other, better options.
I couldn't risk it.
I knew this wouldn't fly, and would be translated as "She's fired".
The husband, a very nice guy, took one more pass at me.
He said, "How about you give her one more preview, and if she's as good as she was the first time, you put her back in the rotation?"
I pondered this for a moment, and said "Let's suppose I do what you say.
And let's say she is as good as she was the first time.
What assurance can you give me that she won't be just as bad as she was the second time when the reviewers are there?"
He said, quite succinctly, "None".
So she quit.
Or was fired.
Name your euphemism.

I felt terrible, but, considering that I am basically a whore for my plays, I had no choice.

All of this, of course, delighted the semi-name actress.

There's an interesting footnote.

Weeks later, I was rehearsing a replacement cast one afternoon at the theatre.
We broke for lunch.
I crossed the street to get to my car.

In the street, I turned to my left, and sitting behind the wheel of her stopped car, along with her young son, was Evelyn.
She was actively scowling at me.

My life flashed before my eyes.
Had she been stalking me?
Was she going to slam her foot on the gas pedal and do me in?

I knew she blamed me.
She never seemed particularly stable, but I never thought she was capable of this.
Nevertheless, I briskly crossed the street, quickly getting out of her range, and never looked back.

So why was she there?
This is a question that to this day has gone unanswered.

*****

So Nice, They Named It Twice.

What I see on TV lately points me towards an increasing inhumanity among humans towards other humans-------
The way BP has treated it's victims, the way Republicans are treating the unemployed, to name just a couple.

What I experienced yesterday points to just the opposite.
And it happened in New York City.
Perhaps the last place anyone might figure that would happen.

I was on one of my Wednesday jaunts from Connecticut to Manhattan to catch a couple of shows.
I bought my first ticket at the TKTS booth in Times Square, and proceeded to the lounge at the Edison Hotel just up the block to sit and wait until show time.

I tried using my new IPhone to get the Internet, but was having some difficulty.
It seems that many indoor facilities have their own Wi-Fi facilities, and in encouraging you to use them (at a fee) block out the Internet reception your IPhone gets ordinarily.
It took me a bit of time and machinations to figure out that this was happening.
Maybe there's a way around this, maybe there isn't.

The best I could do at the moment was to gather up all my paraphernalia and go back outdoors to Times Square, where there was ample seating, and parked myself there, where my IPhone was once again working.

Is anyone out there familiar with the term "Wallet Panic"?

Simply put, it's when you've lost your wallet and can't find it.

I consider the anxiety associated with this condition to be worse than death.

At least when you're dead, you don't care where your wallet is.

I used to put it on a par with "Key Panic", but we all have multiple sets of keys, and Triple A in case we lock our car keys in the car.

There are many addressable solutions to "Key Panic". So it now pales in comparison to "Wallet Panic".

Well, what I experienced yesterday could well have turned into "Wallet Panic".

Instead, because of the humanity of others and the alignment of the stars, it became "Wallet Nirvana".

After being parked out there in Times Square for about fifteen minutes, my IPhone rings.

I answer it:

Caller: Is this Mark?

Me: Yes, this is Mark.

Caller: This is the head of Security at the Edison Hotel. We have your wallet.

Me: I'm just a block away. I'll be right over.

I didn't even know my wallet was missing.

I was spared Wallet Panic.

As I walked briskly back to the Edison, my foremost thought was "How the hell did they know how to reach me?

There was nothing in my wallet that contained my cell phone number.

But, apparently, find it they did.

I seek out the man who called me and identified myself, which wasn't easy, since I didn't have my wallet.

But I answered enough questions satisfactorily to convince him that I was Mark.

He said "Aren't you the least bit curious how we found you?
I responded, "More than the least bit".

Now, this is where the stars, and humanity, all lined up in my favor:
He said "We went through your wallet, and found a check with your name and your wife's name and your Michigan address on it.
We called your local Michigan Long Distance Information.
Your number was listed.
We called it.
Your wife recorded a voicemail message that included 'if you're looking for Mark, this is his cell phone number".

And that's how they found me.

That check had been sitting in my wallet less than a week, and only as a backup check in case anything happened to the one I used to pay for the new IPhone at the A, T, and T store.
And our Michigan phone number just happened to be listed.
And my wife just happened to include my cellphone number in the voicemail message.
And the head of security just happened to go to ALL OF THE TROUBLE to follow through on all of this.
And did it so rapidly that I never experienced Wallet Panic.

I offered him all of the $140 that was in my wallet as a reward.

He wouldn't accept a nickel.

"This is my job. I get paid well for doing my job".

He said this in the gruff manner that New Yorkers are known for.
But that's the key here.
It's just a gruff manner.
That's what the bad rap is against New Yorkers.
As this man proved, and is indicative of the way I believe most New Yorkers are.
That New Yorkers are as nice if not nicer than anybody else.
I'm from there, and I am one, and if anybody wants to argue the point with me, I'll take 'em outside and belt 'em in the mouth.

And that includes you too, lady.

******

The Kid In The Papoose.

While transferring my old Beta tapes to DVDs, I was watching an episode of "Busting Loose".
One of my One-Season Wonders.
Briefly, "Busting Loose" was a gang comedy, contemporarily set in the late 70's.
It was on the order of "Happy Days".
In a rare fit of bravery by CBS, all the characters were Jewish, and unlike Garry Marshall's shows, there was no moral preachiness.
It was only funny.
It kind of broke the ground that was later exploited by "Seinfeld".
We did an episode where the gang of five guys in their early twenties went on a singles resort weekend in the mountains, with one objective: to score with available women.

It was the era of "Charlie's Angels" and "Three's Company", and everything was designed for jiggle.
In this tradition, CBS saw this as an opportunity to fill the screen with voluptuous women in skimpy bathing suits.
As did we, for perhaps less noble reasons, if such a thing was possible.
So fill the screen we did.
Except for one of the women.
The casting person pleaded with me to make a mercy booking for someone who really needed the gig.
She had a two year old child to raise and was having trouble making the rent.
I agreed, basically being a softy at heart.
Even though she really didn't fill out the bathing suit too well.

And, not having anyone to watch her two year old, she dragged her on the set in a papoose that she carried in front of her most of the time, except when she was in a shot, which wasn't often.
She did this without telling anyone she was going to do this beforehand.
So all you saw on the set was this actress, who had a rather unforgettable name, Ildiko Jaid, carrying around this kid in the papoose.
The kid was, truth be told, a little too big to fit in the papoose comfortably.
And Ildiko and the kid were a little difficult to track down during most of the shoot.
You heard a lot of "Where's Ildiko and the kid in the damn papoose?"
Mainly from me.
When she was in the shot, she managed to palm off the kid in the papoose at least momentarily.
Nobody was really dying to watch the kid in the papoose for more than a few minutes at a time.
We gave Ildiko a couple of lines, purely out of sympathy, to up her pay grade.
But, having the opportunity to do it again, I probably wouldn't have.

So making the transfer to DVD, I watched this episode again, I saw Ildiko Jaid again on the screen, still not filling out the bathing suit too well.
Ildiko Jaid is a name you do not forget.
And the Internet being what it is, it was easy for me to satisfy my curiosity about whatever happened to Ildiko Jaid. So I Googled her.
There was nothing under Ildiko Jaid.
But there was something under Ildiko Jaid Barrymore.

I looked up her IMDB entry.
She had been married to John Drew Barrymore.

They had one child in 1975. Only one child.
"Busting Loose" was in 1977.

The kid in the papoose was Drew Barrymore.

Go figure.
I looked at Drew Barrymore's Wikipedia Entry.
It confirmed that Ildiko was her mother.

Who knows what else is out there that I'm not aware
of, and should be?

*****

Dredging Up "The West Point Story".

In the 1950's, James Cagney and Doris Day starred in
two movies together.
Both musicals.
One, in 1955, was the magnificent, stirring, stunning
drama "Love Me Or Leave Me", made at MGM.
It made you wonder why Jimmy and Doris never
made another one together after that.

The other, in 1950, was the dopey, pointless,
ridiculous-on-all-levels musical comedy,
"The West Point Story", turned out by Warner
Brothers.
It made you wonder why Jimmy and Doris ever made
another one together after that.

Cagney, a-mouldering in his grave, probably still has a
backache from the load he had to carry in
"The West Point Story".

I used to see "The West Point Story" on local TV in
New York, all cut up and loaded with commercials,
when I was a kid.
I thought it was out-and-out stupid then.

When the film was made, Cagney, then in his 50's,
played a down-and-out Broadway director who gets
cajoled to go to West Point to direct their annual
show.
Through circumstances that certainly weren't
explained well enough for my young satisfaction, he
had to become a Cadet himself.
And hilarity was supposed to ensue.

The movie didn't make sense on its own terms.

Cagney was supposed to be broke, yet he came up with plane fare (pretty costly in those days) for him and about ten other cadets to go to Washington, then New York City, to satisfy an asinine plot point.
Things like that.
Gordon MacRae was the ingenue male lead.
Lots o' singing.
That didn't hurt or help.
I didn't realize it at the time, but it turns out that most of the songs, by Jule Styne and Sammy Cahn, were taken out of the trunk from a Broadway-bound show in the mid 1940's they did that never got there, called "Gladaseeya!".
But the songs were pretty catchy.
So catchy that they'd stuck in my head.
And, irony of ironies, the movie was extremely watchable.
Primarily because of Cagney.
He worked like a sonofabitch trying to hold the whole thing together.

I recently had the opportunity to catch up with "The West Point Story" because Turner Classic Movies recently ran it, and I Tivoed it and watched it.
This stretches the word "Classic" almost beyond recognition.
It marked the first time I got to see it uncut and without commercials.
It afforded me the opportunity to realize that its senselessness had nothing to do with any cuts that were made.
It was just as senseless uncut.
There were some musical numbers that had been cut, that I saw for the first time.
Some horrendous, others quite dandy.

The quite dandy ones were dance numbers done by Gene Nelson, whom Warner Brothers was grooming to be their Gene Kelly.

Too bad.
They were only off by a few letters.
You might remember him as Will Parker in the film
version of "Oklahoma!"
He was great in that.
And, as I said, dandy in "The West Point Story".

At this point, you might be asking yourself "Why is
this man spending all of this time, and perhaps
wasting all of my time, dredging up a sixty-one-year-
old stinky movie?

If you know me well enough by now, you know I have
my reasons.

Here goes: It was the late 70's.
I was the show runner on one of my one-season
wonders that was about to be cancelled.
I'm sitting in my office.
The phone in my outer office rings.
My secretary answers it.
She puts the caller on hold.
She buzzes me.
I pick up.
"There's a Gene Nelson on the phone. He'd like to talk
to you."
The name was not familiar to her.
Many thoughts went through my head in the brief
moments when I was determining whether or not to
take the call.
Gene Nelson.
It had to be.
THE Gene Nelson. The dancer. The actor.
Why would he be calling me?
He didn't know me.
I didn't know him.
But I had seen his name on lists of available sitcom
directors.
I'd never thought about hiring him.

I'd seen his resume.
He'd directed mostly very soft one-camera sitcoms.
I was doing a hardball three-camera sitcom.
He was obviously calling me to ask for work.

Now, there's nothing wrong with asking anyone for work.
I've been in the position of having to do it myself.
I never did it with a stranger.
Again, nothing wrong with that.

What's wrong is what once happened to me, when the ink wasn't even dry yet on my "She's The Sheriff" contract, and I received a call at home in Ohio from one of the writers I worked with on "Happy Days", a writer whose work never impressed me, and to my knowledge, did not have my home phone number, to ask to be hired on "She's The Sheriff".
This comes under the heading of unfair.
I wasn't afforded the opportunity to not take the call.
Guess what happened?

Back to Gene Nelson.
At this point, there were only a few episodes left on this series, and they were spoken for.
But this was Gene Nelson on the phone.
How many opportunities do I have to talk to Gene Nelson?
And I wouldn't have to blow him off, because I legitimately had no work for him.

So I decided to take the call, and to have fun with him, counting on him to be a good sport, trying to turn this into a not unpleasant experience for both of us.
I guess because I considered myself a fan.

Me: Hello?

Gene: Hi. This is Gene Nelson, I was wondering.....
Me: Wait a minute. THE Gene Nelson?

Gene: Well, I guess you can say......

Me: The star of "The West Point Story"?

Gene is laughing hysterically.

Me: My favorite!

Gene: "The West Point Story"?

Me: Of course!

Gene: Of all the things that I've done, THAT's what you think of?

Me: What else?

Gene: Uh......."Oklahoma!"?

Me: Feh!

Gene is laughing even harder.

Gene: I did "Follies" on Broadway. Did you see that?

Me: Feh! "Give me "The West Point Story".

More laughing from Gene.

I then launch into every song I can think of from "The West Point Story", punctuated by laughter that built and built from Gene.
Gene, by the way, had no songs to sing in the movie.
Only dance numbers.

Me: (Singing, a la Cagney) "B-'postrophe,
K-no postrophe, L-Y-N!
They know my shield, from Ebbets Field to Cheyenne,
You can keep those other places,
Just give me....that oasis,
Where it's earl, not oil,
And a goil's a goil,
And goils are goils at twenty-eight paces........"

"It can only happen in Brooklyn,
On a street called Avenue D,
If you've ever been there,
You'll tell me it's fan-tasy,
But this happened, to me........"

Then I segued into one of Doris Day's
numbers..............
" Ten thousand, four hundred and thirty two sheep
How long can I toss like this?
Ten thousand, four hundred and thirty three sheep
What did you put in that kiss?
I've tried all the remedies
The well-known good advice
Took a hot tub and an alcohol rub
Did the alphabet backwards twice....."

I was hot, so I stuck with Doris for the next number:

"Put your arms around your shoulder
When the order's "Shoulder Arms"
Take a full firm grip of the lady and her charms
If her heart is your objective, you can win it right away
When they play,
The Military Polka.............."

Then I did one that had about four reprises, so it was
done by just about everyone (except Gene):

"You've been kissed I know
In the very last row
When the love scene is on at the movie show
But wait until tonight
And you'll be kissed but right,
By the Kissing Rock........"

I told you the songs were catchy.
And they'd stuck in my head.
You should hear them with Jule Styne's glorious
melodies.

I was pretty much out of gas, and Gene was pretty
much out of breath at that point.
So we got down to the business at hand, which was
pretty much as I expected, and I
'splained the situation.

Gene told me that this was the most entertaining
turndown he'd ever experienced.
I told him that I'd certainly like to think so.

*****

The Charles Lane Moment.

Do you remember Charles Lane?

He was a movie and TV actor..
With, in fact, a far longer career than any other
working actor in the history of show business.
He was around forever.
He was in everything.
He was in "Mr. Smith Goes To Washington".
He was a particular favorite of Frank Capra's.
He was in many of Capra's pictures.
He was in many of EVERYBODY'S pictures.

He was one of those actors you'd recognize instantly,
whether you knew his name or not.
He always played the same type of character: a white-
haired, thin, bespectacled, crotchety, cynical, ornery,
petty, miserly, cantankerous, curmudgeonly,
miserable old geezer.
He even played this character when he was young.
If, in fact, he was ever young.
It never seemed like he was.
Even 77 years ago. When he was in "42nd Street".
His hair was a little darker then.
And he only died two years ago. At 102.

Younger generations probably remember him best as
Homer Bedloe, the white-haired, thin, bespectacled,
crotchety, ornery, petty, miserly, cantankerous,
curmudgeonly, miserable old geezer on "Petticoat
Junction".
"Petticoat Junction" was not a show I had a great deal
of respect for.
I just thought the writing was pretty lazy.
It moved kind of slow. Just like Uncle Joe.
I was not its target audience.

During my second season on "The Odd Couple", we
did an episode where we cast Charles Lane in a
supporting role.
I was in awe.
He was still vigorous.
He would have been about 70.
He looked 95.
He seemed to be living his life in that same crotchety
persona.
That was really him. That's the way he was. It wasn't
acting.
To me, he was a living legend.
I mean, he was in ALL THOSE MOVIES.
He worked with EVERYONE.

The other writers and I were sitting around a table
where later that Wednesday night, after the run-
through rehearsal, we would be doing a rewrite of this
show.
Charles Lane was also there.
We were doing our usual crabbing about how Tony
Randall and Jack Klugman would be at this rewrite
session, overseeing it, and having it result in more
work than we felt would be necessary.
I posited out loud, somewhat sarcastically, "I wonder
if Bea Benaderet would sit around supervising late
night rewrite sessions over at "Petticoat Junction", to
make sure that every word was perfect?"

All of a sudden, Charles Lane, whom I hadn't realized
was within earshot, pipes up with:
"Bea Benaderet was a wonderful woman!
I don't want to hear anything YOU have to say about
Bea Benaderet!"

Now, I never meant to slander Bea Benaderet, whom I thought was a wonderful actress.
Particularly on "The Burns and Allen Show".

I was merely slamming "Petticoat Junction", and indirectly, Jack and Tony.
Charles Lane didn't see that distinction. And probably didn't want to hear "Petticoat Junction" get slammed either.
He probably didn't give a rat's ass about Jack or Tony.
I immediately apologized, telling him that I had nothing but the highest regard for Ms. Benaderet.
Apology was not accepted.
I had pissed off Charles Lane.
When we did the show that Friday night, he was instantly recognized, and he got well deserved applause on his entrance and opening line.
I was very pleased for him.

And I had been given my own Charles Lane white-haired, thin, bespectacled, crotchety, ornery, petty, cantankerous, curmudgeonly, miserable moment, directed solely at me on that Wednesday night.
I cherish it, and wouldn't trade it for anything in the world.

*****

The Robin Ventura Moment.

As I'm writing this, it is opening day for the 2010
Baseball Season.

I have my DirecTV Baseball Package, which allows me
to see all the games, and therefore be selective about
which ones I bet on, as I don't really root for any
particular team.

I try to approach the game with some semblance of
science with regard to betting.
It's a way to prove that I am smarter than the
oddsmakers.
I'm usually fairly successful.
But I did not have an auspicious debut.
I went 0 and 4.
This happens. It's a long season.
But there are different kinds of winning and different
kinds of losing.

There are "Boat Races", which are the most painless
types of winning and losing.
The kinds of games that are pretty much decided by
the third inning.
Either in terms of who is going to win, or in the case of
Total Runs bets, if enough runs are scored.
All that's left is to pray for a rainout, which would
negate the outcome.
Or that it stays dry if you bet the Over.
Boat Races can easily be sloughed off. You win some,
you lose some.

The other kinds of winning and losing are known as
"Nutcutters".
Nutcutters are games where your chances of winning
in the eighth inning are so good, you're already
counting the money.
And then you blow it.

Or your chances are miniscule in the eighth inning,
and somehow you pull it out.
Or you get victimized by circumstance, like an
umpire's bad call.
It is a quite descriptively accurate term.
You literally feel like your nuts were cut off.

Well, I just experienced two Boat Races and two
Nutcutters.
All of which went against me.

The Boat Races involved betting against a pitcher who
had a no-hitter going into the eighth inning.
What are you going to do?
The other involved betting against a team that jumped
out to an 8-0 lead in the third inning and held it.
What are you going to do?

The Nutcutters involved backing a team (Kansas City)
that was an underdog, getting good odds, with a 5-0
lead in the eighth inning, that let the other team
(Detroit) score 6 in the bottom of the 8th to beat me,
6-5.
I threw things at the screen.
Soft things, like pillows.
Based on past experience, my wife doesn't allow me
any items in the room that can break things.

This was shortly followed by blowing a Total Runs bet
where I bet that the two teams, the Yankees and the
Angels, would score a combined total of less than 11
runs.
It was 5-0 Yankees going into the 8th.
Things looked promising.

7-1 going into the 9th. Still pretty optimistic.
Then, the Angels went on enough of a tear in the 9th
to make it 7-5, and pick my pocket.
More flying soft objects.
Back-to-back Nutcutters.

But hardly the worst Nutcutter I ever experienced.
Far worse pickpocketing went on during one occasion
more than ten years ago.

It was the sixth game of the 2000 National League
Championship Series between the New York Mets and
the Atlanta Braves at Shea Stadium.
I had a Total Runs bet.
I took the Over.
The number was 9 1/2.
I needed 10 runs to be scored to win. 9 would lose.
It was the bottom of the 9th. 4-3, Braves.

The Mets loaded the bases.
I was down to praying for a walk to tie the game and
keep it going, or a wild pitch to tie the game, or a not
so solid base hit to tie the game.
And then I could still easily lose.
I'd need the Braves to score more than one run in
extra innings to have a chance.
But in this bottom of the 9th inning, as soon as the
winning run crosses the plate, the game is over.
Not many viable options there. If that runner scores
from second, I'm dead.

My only real prayer was for a Grand Slam Home Run.
A Home Run is the exception to the rule.
When there is a Home Run, all baserunners score.
That would get me to 11. Enough to win.

Robin Ventura was at bat for the Mets.
It got to a full count and a lot of fouling off of pitches
by Ventura, and a lot of plotzing by me.
But that was only the preliminary plotzing.
What followed was the unfathomable:

Ventura hits a towering blast over the Right Field
wall.
A Grand Slam.
My prayer was answered.

I win.
Ventura is immediately mobbed by the fans as he
rounds first base.
I'm jumping up and down like a lunatic.
Ventura tries to keep running, but the fans won't let
him.

The Official Scorers, having the option to do this,
decide to award Ventura a single.
The runners score from third and second base.
The Mets win 5-4.
I lose.
If Ventura had merely been allowed to trot around the
bases, which was his God-given right,
I would have won.
But he couldn't.
So I lost.
My nuts were sliced and diced.
I still can't function.

Those Official Scorers and those fans did a better job
than Benny the Dip.

*****

Making Friends Wherever I Go.

I'm in Connecticut this week, planning to make a
Wednesday jaunt into Manhattan to catch a couple of
shows.
Last time out, I saw "Race", what turned out to be a
truly great David Mamet play.
I recommend it to all.
But my comment has to do with what happened
before the curtain went up, and at intermission.

I was in my seat in the orchestra, and behind me was
this group of people who knew each other and were
talking to each other.
One of them was this old Jewish guy named Harry.
I knew this because he looked old, had a heavy Jewish
accent, and one of the others kept calling him "Harry".
So I'm sitting there, and one of Harry's colleagues says
"So, Harry, did you see 'Superior Donuts'?"
"Superior Donuts" is a play by the author of
"August Osage County". No slouch.

Harry says "Yeah, I saw it. Piece of shit.
I don't know why I wasted my time."

Now, I saw "Superior Donuts". It was a wonderful
play. Involving, gut-wrenching, funny, well played.
But according to Harry, a piece of shit.

I don't say anything.
Everyone's entitled to his opinion.
Maybe not quite as loud as Harry, but still entitled.

The same colleague then says "What about 'Wishful
Drinking', Harry? Did you see that?"

"Wishful Drinking" was Carrie Fisher's one-woman
autobiographical show. I saw that, too.
Now, to be fair, I am an unabashed fan of Carrie
Fisher.

She's a great writer, wit, and storyteller. And all of these skills were on display in "Wishful Drinking".

Not according to Harry. "Yeah, I sat through that crap. Only because I was stuck in the middle of the row and couldn't leave after five minutes.
All she does is talk about herself."

I'm pretty sure that everyone else who saw that show knew going in that this show was autobiographical in nature, which would give her at least some license to talk about herself.

I don't say anything.

Then, about five minutes before the curtain goes a up, a large woman enters the row in front of mine.
A large buxom woman. With purple tinged hair. Showing a lot of cleavage. Showing off a large tattoo on her largely exposed left breast.

From behind me, I hear Harry say to one of his colleagues "You know what I'll bet her name is?"
"What, Harry?" replies his colleague/straight-man.
"I'll bet her name is June", replies Harry. "You know why?"
"Why, Harry?" replies the hyphenate.
"Because she's busting out all over", says Harry, who then has an uncontrollable fit of laughter.
Now this is not necessarily the worst joke in the world, but in Harry's hands, it sure came close.

And, of course, everyone finds it endearing when someone laughs hysterically at his own jokes.
I don't say anything.

The curtain goes up, and I am treated to one of the greatest first acts in theatrical history.
The audience practically gives the first act a standing ovation.
The lights come up.

From behind me, I hear the hyphenate ask
"So what do you think, Harry?"
Harry says "I don't even know why I bother to leave
the house anymore"
Given my limited but growing knowledge of Harry, I
was inclined to agree with him.
"This thing isn't going anywhere. It stinks."

NOW, I decide to say something. I turn around and
face Harry.

ME: Okay. "Superior Donuts" was a piece of shit.
"Wishful Drinking" was crap. This show stinks.
"June is busting out all over", by you, is hilarious.

I turn back around.

HARRY (slowly and deliberately, to my back) Was I
talking to you? Would I ever, in my wildest dreams,
ever talk to you? What gives you the right to talk to me
like that?

ME: (turning back around to face Harry) Because
you've subjected yourself to me and this entire side of
the theater!

I turned back around, the curtain went back up, I saw
an even better second act, and that was the end of it.

I made sure that was the end of it by standing up
immediately during the ovation, showing Harry that I
was, in fact, six feet six inches tall and 250 pounds, in
case he was still in a fight-picking mood.
He wasn't.

Sometimes I think that maybe I should apply for an
Ambassadorship.

******

Things That Should Be Done In Your House.

I reminded myself today of something I had witnessed many years ago.
Something that made me laugh really hard when it happened.
Maybe it will make you laugh too.

It was during my show running days at Paramount on one of the sitcoms.
It was one of those rare nights when we worked late enough to start getting really hungry, but got done early enough to be unable to justify ordering in dinner for the writers and myself.

This only occurred rarely, and when it did, the writers were, as one, crestfallen.
Because this meant they had to buy their own dinners.

Four of us decided to go out for some Chinese food.
We went to a pretty good local joint near the studio.

When you order Chinese food in a restaurant, there are two ways to go:
You order individually, or you order "family style", with everyone sharing each dish.

If you're Jews, you order family style.
I've never seen my tribe do it any other way.
What is it about Jews and Chinese food?
We can't get enough of it.
Yet I can't, for the life of me, ever recall seeing a Chinese person eating Jewish food.... Oh well.....

So the four of us are there, and we decide to let one of us, Bernie, do the ordering.

We do this because he is a much more finicky eater than the rest of us, and usually orders well, usually by being very specific about how the food should be prepared.

And the food usually came out better that way.
We trusted in Bernie.

The ancient, frail Chinese waiter came to our table.

Bernie launches into his order-----

Bernie: First, we'd like a tureen of Won Ton Soup, as hot as you can make it.....

Waiter: (Writing on his checkpad) Hot as you can make it.....

Bernie: Crispy noodles in the soup, not on the side.

Waiter: But we always bring on the side.

Bernie: In the soup. Not on the side.

Waiter: (As he is writing)......not on the side.

Bernie: An order of Subgum Fried Wonton.

Waiter: (Writing) Subgum Fried Wonton.

Bernie: And make sure the Won Ton is extra crispy.

Waiter: (Writing) Extra Crispy.

Bernie: Right.

Waiter: You want noodles soggy but Won Ton extra crispy?

Bernie: That's right. We'd also like an order of Shrimp and Lobster Sauce.

Waiter: (Writing)....Shrimp and Lobster Sauce.

Bernie: But no egg yolk in the lobster sauce.

Waiter (Staring, then writing)....no egg yolk.

Bernie: Egg white is fine, but no egg yolk.

Waiter: (Writing furiously, and I mean furiously)....egg white fine, no egg yolk.

Bernie: An order of Beef Lo Mein.

Waiter: (Writing)...Beef Lo Mein.

Bernie: But make the noodles as firm as possible.

Waiter: Other noodles soggy, these noodles firm?

Bernie: That's right.

Waiter: But Lo Mein noodles always soggy.

Bernie: That's true. But here, they make them TOO soggy. So I want them firm.

Waiter: (Writing) Too soggy...want them firm.

Bernie: An order of Mu Shoo Pork.

Waiter: (Writing, with pen poised to await further instructions)....Mu Shoo Pork........

Bernie: Make sure the Plum Sauce is on the side, not on it.

Waiter: (Writing) On the side, not on it.

Bernie: You know what? Make that Moo Shoo Chicken.

Waiter: (Tearing up the check and about to storm off) Eat in your house!!!

The waiter is now gone.

We all look at each other.

I'm stifling the biggest giggle I've ever had in me.

Bernie: Should we try someplace else?

Me: We'd better. If they make him come back and take the order again, you know he's going to take a piss in the Won Ton Soup.

So we left, and, no longer in the mood, we went out for Burgers.

Just thought I'd share.

*****

Dr. Rothman, Tune Detective.

In Neil Simon's wonderfully funny play and movie,
"The Sunshine Boys", early on, the following exchange
takes place between Willie Clark and Al Lewis, the old
vaudevillians based on the real comedy team, Smith
and Dale.
It takes place in Willie's apartment, as the two of them
are sitting, drinking tea.

Now, this is from memory, won't be totally accurate,
and is most likely condensed.
But you should get the gist.

Willie: You know Sol Burton died?

Al: Go on....Who's Sol Burton?

Willie: You don't remember Sol Burton?

Al: .....oh yes. The manager from the Belasco Theatre.

Willie: That was Sol Bernstein.

Al: No, not Sol Bernstein. Sol BURTON was the
manager from the Belasco.

Willie: Sol BERNSTEIN was the manager from the
Belasco, and it wasn't the Belasco, it was the Morosco.

Al: Sid WEINSTEIN was the manager from the
Morosco. Sol BURTON was the manager from the
Belasco. Sol BERNSTEIN I don't know who the hell he
was. Wait a minute. Wasn't Sid Weinstein the
songwriter?

Willie: No for Chrissakes! That's SOL BURTON!

Al: The one who wrote "Lady, Lady Be My Baby"?

Willie: That's what I'm telling you! Sol Burton! The lousy songwriter.

Al: Oh, THAT Sol Burton.....He died?

Willie: Last week.

Al: Where?

Willie: In "Variety".

Al: Sure, now I remember. He rhymed "Lady" with "Baby". No wonder he's dead.

"No wonder he's dead". One of the great lines.

Now, this begs the very logical question:
"Should the Death Penalty be applied to bad song-writing?"
I suppose not.

But should it be applied to song plagiarism?'
The jury is starting to come in on this one, closely following the Laws of Nature.

Some examples:

In 1955, in one of his rarer solo endeavors, Johnny Mercer wrote music and lyrics for the movie "Daddy Longlegs" In it, he scored a major hit with a song called "Something's Gotta Give".

The very next year, in one of his far too common solo endeavors, Steve Allen wrote music and lyrics to "This Could Be The Start of Something Big'".
Probably his biggest hit.
And he didn't have many.

Same subject matter, same chord structure, same tempo.

Steve Lawrence and Eydie Gorme recorded both
songs, and if I'm not mistaken, used the same
orchestral charts for both.

They're the same song.

In the early 40's, Duke Ellington wrote the classic
"Don't Get Around Much Anymore".
In the mid- 70's, Joe Raposo was primarily known for
the songs he wrote for "Sesame Street".
"It's Not Easy Bein Green" etc.
He then wrote the theme song for the TV series
"Three's Company".
With a slightly perkier tempo, musically, it's "Don't
Get Around Much Anymore".
Joe Raposo died at 52.
I'm just sayin' .

There were a couple of major lawsuits regarding song
plagiarism.
Ronald Mack, the writer of "He's So Fine", a song
recorded by the girl group "The Chiffons", sued
George Harrison for plagiarism when Harrison came
out with "My Sweet Lord".
A direct steal attempt, and Harrison was easily thrown
out at second base.
He paid a hefty fine.
The Chiffons, capitalizing on the lawsuit, then came
out with their own recording of "My Sweet Lord".
What a sick business.

There was another lawsuit.
Mack David, a songwriter of note, sued Jerry Herman
because a song David had written in 1948, and had
some success with, called "Sunflower", shared many
of the same notes of the first four bars of "Hello
Dolly!"

Now, I've heard "Sunflower", and we've all heard
"Hello Dolly!"

Take my word for it, "Hello Dolly!" is a MUCH better
song than "Sunflower".
Louis Armstrong would never have recorded
"Sunflower".
And it's not very similar.
And Herman, maintaining that he had never heard of
"Sunflower", wanted to challenge it in court.
But those involved in the show "Hello Dolly!"
persuaded Herman to settle out of court, for the good
of the show, which he reluctantly did.
Jerry Herman certainly got a bad rap there.

In the late 50's, Chuck Berry wrote the great "Sweet
Little Sixteen".

In the early 60's, Brian Wilson wrote "Surfin U.S.A."
for the Beach Boys.

It's the same song.

The late Cy Coleman holds the record, as far as I
know. Whether intentional or not.

In 1940, songwriters Matt Dennis and Tom Adair
wrote a song called "Everything Happens To Me."
It was quite popular. Sinatra recorded it.

In 1952, Cy Coleman wrote a song called "Why Try To
Change Me Now?"'
Sinatra had success with that one, too.

It was "Everything Happens To Me" sideways.

Cy Coleman wrote a song called "If They Could See
Me Now", for the musical "Sweet Charity".
It has been pointed out by others than myself that it is
"Waitin' For The Robert E. Lee" sideways.

Shortly before his death, Coleman came out with a
really wonderful CD, where he sang his own songs.

I've always been a sucker for composers singing their own songs. And he was one of the best at it.
On this CD, there was a fairly new song that he had written and performed, called "I Really Love You".
It is, virtually note for note, with the same tempo, Frankie Valli's "My Eyes Adored You", which, of course, contains the sledgehammer lyric of all time: "Though I never laid a hand on you, My eyes adored you".

Cy Coleman also indulged in stealing from himself.
For the show "The Will Rogers Follies", a show I absolutely loved, he wrote a song called "Hooray For Our Favorite Son" for Keith Carradine and a long line of chorus girls to perform, sitting down, all of them having straw hats.
It was performed Rockettes-style with great Tommy Tune choreography.
It regularly brought down the house.
But if you are able to look past the chorus girls and the straw hats, you might notice that the song is essentially a speeded up version of Coleman's hit song for Peggy Lee several years earlier, called "Pass Me By".

Even the great Irving Berlin stole from himself.
For the revival of "Annie Get Your Gun" in 1966, he wrote a new song, a contrapuntal duet for Ethel Merman and her co-star Bruce Yarnell, called "Old Fashioned Wedding".
It's essentially another version of the contrapuntal duet "You're Just In Love" from Berlin's "Call Me Madam", also starring Merman.
In fact, all 4 parts can be sung at the same time, using the same orchestration.

Just a couple of days ago, my wife and I, in the car, were listening to the Sinatra station on Sirius Radio.
A Sinatra song came on, a rarity in that I had never heard it before.

It was called something like "To Be In Love".
It was certainly never a hit, or I would have heard of it.
But what it was, and this is how I expressed it to my wife, was "Young At Heart" sideways.

"Young at Heart" was a huge hit for Sinatra. It was pleasant, upbeat, with a very interesting dissonant chord in it, that gave it a lot more depth.
This other song had the exact same orchestration, with the same dissonant chord in the same place.
I'd bet anything that when "Young at Heart" was released as a single, this other song was on the flip side.

Anthony Newley wrote "Feelin' Good" for the only black cast member of "The Roar of The Greasepaint, The Smell of The Crowd"
It was merely a much more somber version of Gershwin's "It Ain't Necessarily So".
From "Porgy and Bess". Written for a black singer.

Even the great Stephen Sondheim indulged in thievery, although he is so knowledgeable about musical history that he probably considered it homage.
There's a song in Sondheim's "Company" called "Poor Baby".
The underscoring and much of the melody is Gershwin's Piano prelude No. 2.
Listen to them one after another, and see what you think.

So what have we learned from all this?

Steve Allen----dead.

Joe Raposo----dead.

George Harrison----dead.

Cy Coleman-----dead.

Anthony Newley---dead.

Irving Berlin----dead. (All right, he'd probably be about 120 now, so maybe that isn't fair).

The guy who ripped off "Young at Heart----it was so long ago that he's probably dead.

Frank Sinatra, who had a great ear, and must have known what was going on with the "Young at Heart" ripoff, and "Why Try to Change Me Now?"-----dead.

Jerry Herman-----has been dealing with the HIV virus for about 15 years----still alive.

It appears that Nature has provided Justice.

I don't hold out much hope for Brian Wilson, or Sondheim.

This from last Christmas-----------

One of the few things I like about the Christmas season which we're in right now, and there aren't many, is the onslaught of Christmas songs on the radio.
Not the Carols.
The hit records that were made over the years, that only show up in November and December on the airwaves.

I love 'em all.
And I love the seasonality of their appearance.
I love the sense of history involved in hearing them.

Two weeks ago, my wife and I were in the car, listening to a radio station that was playing all the old ones.

They played Burl Ives singing "Have a Holly Jolly Christmas".
It brought a smile to my face, and my head was bobbin' up and down in rhythm.

This was immediately followed by Brenda Lee singing "Rockin' Around The Christmas Tree"
Also a favorite.

In the middle of Brenda's second chorus, something occurred to me, that had never occurred to me before: "Holly Jolly Christmas" and "Rockin' Around The Christmas Tree" are THE SAME SONG!

By the same song, I don't mean note for note. But the same chord structure and musical progression.

You could have had Burl and Brenda standing up there on the same stage, with one orchestra playing the same accompaniment, each singing their own song, in the same tempo, and it would have been perfect counterpoint.

Am I, as usual, the last person in the world to notice this?
And if so, why did it take me all this time?

I tried to impress my wife with this discovery, and, of course, she couldn't have cared less.

A few days later, we were back in the car, listening to the same station, and after a few songs, they played Gene Autry singing "Rudolph The Rednosed Reindeer".

I had another epiphany. "Rudolph" was ALSO THE SAME SONG!

You could have thrown Gene up there on the same stage with Burl and Brenda, and it would be three part counterpoint!

I missed that one too!

My wife was still less than impressed.

That night, I went to Wikipedia. It turns out that all three songs were written by the same person. Johnny Marks.
These were his three biggest hits.

It got me to thinking, and as I kept hearing Christmas standards on the radio, I kept hearing
OTHER songs that were this SAME SONG!

"Frosty The Snowman". Throw Jimmy Durante up on the stage with Burl, Brenda, and Gene.
Four part counterpoint.

"Walking in a Winter Wonderland".
Throw Johnny Mathis up there too.
Five part counterpoint.

"Jingle Bell Rock".
Shlep Bobby Helms up there too.
Six part Counterpoint.

This stage is getting pretty crowded.

"It's Beginning to Look a Lot Like Christmas", "Here Comes Santa Claus", "Melekelikemaka, the Hawaiian Christmas Song"----toss up Perry, Elvis, and Bing and the Andrews Sisters.
They're all now standing shoulder to shoulder.

Nine part counterpoint. All the same song.

Before you think I've gone completely off the deep end, I racked my brain to come up with Christmas standards that WEREN'T this same song.
And there are plenty of them:

Chestnuts Roasting on an Open Fire (The Christmas Song)
White Christmas
The Little Drummer boy
All I want for Christmas is My Two Front Teeth
I'm Gettin' Nuttin' for Christmas
I Saw Mommy Kissing Santa Claus
Blue Christmas (although even that one is close)
Santa Baby
Sleigh Ride
Santa Claus is Comin to Town
Felis Navidad
It's the Most Wonderful Time of the Year
The Chipmunks Christmas Song
Grandma Got Run Over By a Reindeer
Let it Snow
Silver Bells
The Christmas Waltz (Sinatra)
I'll Be Home for Christmas
Have Yourself a Merry Little Christmas

These songs aren't the same song as the other nine.
As far as I can tell, none are the same as each other, or anything else.

So it's not me.

It's too bad that so many of the singers who would have filled the stage with the nine part counterpoint are gone now.

I'd have paid a pretty penny to see them all do it.

Merry Christmas to all, and I'll see you next week, when this whole thing blows over.

*****

Why I Love Ted Turner.

I must say that the first time I encountered Ted Turner on TV, when he was being interviewed, I was less than impressed, to say the least.

With his somewhat lisping drawl, and rather vacant look, he reminded me of O.Z. Whitehead, a great character-actor and member of John Ford's stock company ("The Grapes of Wrath", The Man Who Shot Liberty Valance", etc.), who had a lisping drawl, and a rather vacant look.

Perhaps the height of O.Z. Whitehead's work was in Ford's "The Last Hurrah", which starred Spencer Tracy as the corrupt but well-intended Mayor of Boston, who was seeking re-election one last time.

This is a great movie, and one of my favorites. (These two things can sometimes be mutually exclusive.)

Whitehead played the son of one of Tracy's adversaries, a banker who is deliberately holding out on a loan for public works that Tracy was counting on. The banker was played by Basil Rathbone.

In an attempt to embarrass Rathbone into giving him the loan, Tracy secretly invites Whitehead to his office to offer him the job of Fire Commissioner, knowing that Whitehead would be in way over his head, and fail miserably.

It's a hilarious scene. Whitehead is extremely flattered. "Fire Commithioner?", he asks.

It culminates with Tracy placing a big fireman's hat on Whitehead's head. Whitehead is tickled at the prospect, and Tracy has one of his flunkies take a photograph of Whitehead with the Fireman's hat on his head, looking ridiculous.

Tracy then takes the photograph to Rathbone, who, knowing he's been successfully blackmailed, reluctantly grants Tracy the loan.

So the first reaction I had upon seeing Ted Turner was "He's the Fire Commithioner!"

Shortly after that, Turner, who owned the Atlanta Braves baseball team, decided to fire his manager, and become the manager himself. This lasted, I think, a day.

In my eyes, seeing Turner in his Powder-Blue Atlanta Braves road uniform, he had officially become the Fire Commithioner.

But first (and second) impressions can be incredibly deceiving.

Aside from being a brilliant businessman (Everything Trump wants to be), he is responsible for more positive changes in our daily lives than anyone else:

1) He created the Superstation.

He took a TV station that he owned, a UHF station no less, and figured out that it could be hooked up to a satellite and be able to broadcast all over the place. He put his Atlanta Braves' games on the Superstation. Do you have any idea what this means to a baseball fan who lives in the boondocks, where no other baseball is broadcast?
Or a baseball fan who lives anywhere else?
It's one more game a day to watch and bet on.
This spawned copycats.
WOR in New York started showing the Mets' games.
WGN in Chicago still shows most of the Cubs' games.
And the Cubs still play most of their home games in the daytime.
When NOBODY ELSE is playing.

What a blessing for out-of-work, shut-in baseball bettors (excuse me, I meant fans.).

2) He invented CNN.

CNN, with its 24/7 news cycle, has single-handedly changed the way news is broadcast on TV.
It has made the major network nightly news broadcasts virtually obsolete.
It has spawned wonderful competition from MSNBC.
And, of course, terrible competition from, God help us, Fox News.
I think I'm starting to let my political leanings show.

The only times you really need Network news are on major holidays, when CNN runs nothing but interview reruns, usually Larry King, and MSNBC runs nothing but old shows about prisons and rape.
As much as you want.
And Fox News brings you, well, Fox News.
The only place you get REALLY fair-and-balanced news on Christmas Day is on the nightly network news broadcast.
And you don't get Brian Williams, either.
Usually you get Lester Holt.

Ted is unquestionably THE Innovator.

3) Turner Classic Movies.

Probably, pound for pound, the best channel on your Cable or Satellite package.
There are now generations that not only don't notice it, but if they do, have no idea what a breakthrough it has been.
Before TCM, there was no such thing as an uncut, non-commercial-interrupted movie shown on Television.
And TCM's inventory is astounding.
Films I didn't even know existed.

When I was growing up in New York, there was the
next best thing----
"The Million Dollar Movie."
Shown on WOR, channel 9, the same channel that
grew up to be a Superstation, it was on like eleven
times a week.
And what it did was show a Classic---- Citizen Kane,
Casablanca, King Kong, The Hunchback of Notre
Dame, The Jolson Story----
One movie, eleven times in one week.
And you'd watch it over and over.
It was like going to Film School.

I explained this to a movie-fanatic friend of mine, who
grew up in Portsmouth Ohio, where, with rabbit ears,
he was only able to get three snowy channels out of
Columbus.
He is also one of the few who remembers Sammy
Davis singing "Ee-o-ee-leven" in "Ocean's Eleven".
His only source for seeing Hollywood feature film
product was on something called "The Early Show,
with Flippo the Clown".
From what I understand, not the best way to see a
movie.
Flippo was this guy, dressed up as a clown, in full
clown makeup, who considered himself just as much
of the entertainment as the movie.
Aside from commercials, during breaks he would sing
songs, play "Dialing For Dollars", announce his
upcoming Car-Dealership-Opening appearances, a lot
of times not giving a hoot about getting back to the
movie.
My ex-wife also grew up in Portsmouth.
I was introduced to her by the movie-fanatic friend.
Something he still apologizes to me for.
She also grew up on Flippo.
Any time we'd talk about some old movie, she'd
usually say "Oh, yeah. I saw that on 'Flippo'. "

By the end of our marriage, we were living in Columbus, a production of one of my plays in Columbus was being planned, and casting was underway.

Everyone involved thought the guy who played Flippo would be ideal for one of the key roles, and they were right.

So he came over to my house, and we adjourned to my basement to go over the dialogue.

After a few minutes, my now ex-wife, who at that point showed virtually no interest in my career (one of the major problems), descended the stairs, and in one of the most endearing moments of our marriage, introduced herself to Flippo.

In under a minute I got to witness a 33-year-old adult melt into a 9-year-old.

When I told my friend about "Million Dollar Movie", he was astounded.

He said "No wonder you know so much more about movies than I do!! All I had was Flippo!!"

But "Million Dollar Movie" can't hold a candle to Turner Classic Movies.

Another channel, American Movie Classics, tried to give TCM a run for its money, but it finally succumbed to having commercial breaks.

The first runner-up is the Fox Movie Channel, which is a close second, but they show too many Cinemascope movies in pan-and scan form.

TCM has spoiled me and made this unacceptable.

TCM is a Godsend. And Ted Turner is the God who sent it.

4) Colorized Movies. Ted Turner was and is one of its main supporters and proponents.

I know they've kind of fallen by the wayside, but perhaps they'll make a comeback.

And I know that there are a lot of naysayers about them, but I consider Colorized Movies to be Miracles of Nature. A great invention.

Right up there with Edison, and the Wright Brothers.

The putter-downers, Frank Capra, Jimmy Stewart, Woody Allen, and almost every member of the Directors Guild (I may be the only holdout) consider it a travesty.
"It's not the way we intended our movies to be seen" was the pooh-poohing, whining, and general outcry.

Let me put it this way: Where was the hue and cry when all these old movies started showing up on Early TV?
On little screens. Cut up. With lots of commercials in-between.
A lot of them were movies that were made in color, but only able to be seen in Black and White.
As far as I know, these people quietly took the residual money they were getting, and kept their mouths shut.

To me, it boils down to how good a paint job it is.

Ever see the Colorized "Yankee Doodle Dandy"?
A far better movie. I think the only reason it was made in Black-and White is that Jack Warner was too cheap to shoot it in color.

Maybe some movies stand it better than others.
But we live in an age where entire generations won't watch anything in Black-And-White.
Anything except "I Love Lucy".

So if colorizing the classics, even "Citizen Kane", means a significantly larger audience for them in the future, I say let's have at it.

And this is why I love Ted Turner.
*****

Cheek.

It means "Totally self-absorbed nerve".

The Yiddish word is "Chutzpah". But there is a certain charm attached to "Chutzpah".

"Cheek" is a less charitable term. It's what an anti-semite would call someone with "Chutzpah".

Cheek has much more of an "immodest" element to it.

I guess a case could be made that anyone that has his own blog and sounds off on a daily basis has "Cheek".

It's not necessarily a good case.
Not to say I'm not somewhat self-absorbed. I am.
I'm also very immodest in some areas, and very modest in most.
This blog was virtually handed to me.
I received a pop-up from AOL saying "Start your own Blog. It's free. Just go here, and push a few buttons".
My wife had been after me for a while to start my own website, and to write more.
But I, being computer-illiterate, thought the procedure too complicated.
She'd say "We can get a guy to set it up for you".
I thought paying some guy for the privilege of being able to mouth off to whatever segment of the world that was out there for me just smacked of "Cheek".
We both just let the idea go.
Then I received the AOL pop-up.
It just became too easy. I didn't have to go out of my way to impose my way to the public's heart.

I had never been an essayist. I had no idea whether I'd be any good at it.
But the price was right to try it.
And I knew I had stories to tell.

If nobody was reading, or I received more negative reaction than positive (blog-readers are not shy), I would have performed an early abortion. To continue would be cheeky. And I prefer to think of myself as not that.
But it turns out that many more than nobody was reading. And more and more than nobody all the time.
And the reaction has been overwhelmingly positive.
So, in this case: Cheek? I plead innocent. And I think I have the right to point fingers.

I'll offer up a couple of examples of what I consider "Cheek".

In 1979, the actress Phyllis Newman appeared in a brief run of a one-woman musical, "The Madwoman Of Central Park", on Broadway.
I'm sure she would have liked it to be more than brief.

She was best known as a game-show panelist, talk show guest, starring in short-run musicals, closed-out-of-town-before-opening musicals, replacement for other actresses in long-running Broadway musicals, being married to the great lyricist Adolph Green, and winning a Tony Award as Best Supporting Actress in a Musical, for "Subways Are For Sleeping", where she beat out Barbra Streisand in "I Can Get It For You Wholesale".
I saw both shows. It was highway robbery.
But she was certainly not an untalented woman.

Being married to Green, she hung out with the creme de la creme of chi-chi New York show biz.
She got to call Leonard Bernstein "Lennie", Lauren Bacall "Betty", Stephen Sondheim "Steve", etc.

In a biography of Judy Holliday, an incident is described.

Judy has been invited to a party at the Green's. The guest of honor was Peter Sellers.
She arrives, rings the doorbell, Phyllis Newman opens the door and announces, in the most sombre tones, "Peter Sellers cannot come".
To which Judy immediately replies, musically, "Ee-yi-ee-yi-o!"
I'm guessing Phyllis didn't find this funny.

So I'm in New York one weekend, looking to catch up on Broadway shows, and I see that her one-woman show is playing.
I had no idea what this show was about, nor was there any indication in the advertising.
I just figured she invented this character, and found a hook to play her in a one-woman musical.
But my ever-trusty shit detector said "Not worth the money". So I spent it on other shows, with no regrets.

About six months later, I'm back in California.
The show long closed, PBS presents a performance of "The Madwoman of Central Park West" on TV.

This time, I figure the price is right. So I watch.
A good twenty minutes into it, after a couple of songs, one I'd never heard, and one I knew from another Broadway show, I still had no idea what this show was about, or why it existed.

Then, she started talking about appearing on game-shows, and talk shows, being married to Adolph Green, and knowing Lennie and Betty and Steve.
And dealing with the delivery boys from Gristede's, the local Manhattan "hoo-hah" food market, and what a tough life it could be sometimes.

Aaahhh! It's a musical autobiography.
About a life that very few people can relate to.
Now, there's nothing wrong with doing a musical autobiography.

Lena Horne did one. So did Peggy Lee.
But, come on. Phyllis Newman ain't no Lena Horne or
Peggy Lee.
And she was charging the same prices.
But that's not the point. The point is:
Isn't there some sort of moral obligation to let the
potential audience know that a musical autobiography
is what you're doing, and not surprise them with that
fact during the performance?
An obligation to let them decide whether or not they
find your life interesting enough to be musicalized
before they shell out their good money to see it?
She didn't feel this obligation. She just assumed an
audience would be dying to see it.
It probably did not even occur to her that they
wouldn't.

This is "Cheek".

Even Suzanne Somers, who brought this apparently
really crummy show of hers to Broadway, and got
laughed off the street, was honest enough to let you
know that what you were in for, and being charged an
arm and a leg for, was autobiographical.

"Madwoman" was not an unentertaining show. It was
not terrible. At home. In my house.
In California. On PBS. For free.   .

But if my shit detector had failed me, and I had spent
good money to see it, I'm sure that at intermission, I
would have left the theatre, headed for the nearest
fruitstand, returned with a bag of tomatoes, and
thrown them at her from my seat.
And that couldn't have led to anything productive.

It's a good thing for all concerned that I saw it in
California, in my easy-chair.
Far away from tomato-throwing distance.

Next case: This one will be another Essay-a-clef.

In this case, I just don't want to make this big an enemy.

I think it's another great example of Cheek.

Now, I got this story second-hand from one of the eyewitnesses, who is a very reliable source,
and I was around, and recall seeing the parties involved, but not the incident itself.

When I lived near Lake Tahoe in the 90's, I spent most evenings at Caesar's Tahoe, which has since changed hands and is known as something else. I don't remember what.

Every year, in June, Caesar's Tahoe held a major Pro-Am golf tournament.
Lots of celebrities, lots of retired sports greats, and lots of retired sports not-so-greats who were great golfers were in the amateur tournament.
And at night, they were all in the casino, gambling, meeting other guests, having dinner.
I got to meet a lot of my heroes. I got to meet Joe Namath, and chat with him.
He couldn't have been more gracious and charming. It was delightful.

I also rode up the elevator with Joe DiMaggio.
Just me and Joltin' Joe.
I could have asked him where he has gone, but I restrained myself.
True to his image, he seemed very uncomfortable, and looked away from me the whole ride.
Not exactly a Kodak moment.
Even if it was, I wouldn't have had the nerve to put film in the camera.
Now, here's the part I didn't see. It was told to me by a

friend of mine, a woman named Janine, who was the hostess at the Caesar's Tahoe Chinese restaurant.

During one of those tournament weekends, a very well-known Oscar-winning movie director, (Let's call him, appropriately, Oscar) with many big hits under his belt, who won his Oscar for a film that won several Oscars, including Best Picture, and Best Actor, was staying at Caesar's.
(Those are all the clues I'm giving you, except that he won his Oscar before the 90's, and it's not Spielberg or Scorcese)
He was having a rather late dinner with someone who seemed to be his wife (Let's call her Mrs. Oscar) at the Chinese restaurant.
According to Janine, Oscar noticed a lot of the other celebrities finishing their dinners, and not being handed a check.
They were being "comped".

Oscar then decided to order more food. More than the two of them could possibly eat.
Oscar and Mrs. Oscar finished their dinner and asked for doggie-bags for the massive amount of food they didn't eat.
The waiter takes the uneaten food, brings it back in doggie-bags, along with the check.

"What's this?", Oscar asked. "Your check, sir", the waiter responded.
"Why am I getting a check?" Oscar inquired, rather heatedly.

At this point, Janine stepped in. "Is there a problem, sir?"
Mrs. Oscar piped up "Don't you realize who this is?"
"Uh, no" said Janine.

"He's Oscar, that's who". He directed "_____",
and "_____"
Oscar then prompted her "and '_____'."
"Right. And '_____' . He's got an Academy Award
for God sakes".

Janine said "Let me get the manager". She goes off
and gets Doug, the restaurant manager.
Doug is a very sweet man. I used to call him Douggie.
And he didn't mind.

Oscar has steam coming out of his ears.

Douggie goes over to Oscar's table. After he asks
what's wrong, Oscar and the Mrs. go into their plaint,
and the litany of Oscar's credits.
Douggie says, "Do you have a comp slip ?"
Oscar says "Do I really need one?"
Douggie says "Would you like to speak to a Host?"
Mrs. Oscar says "Well, obviously we're getting
nowhere with you!"

Douggie says "I'll have him come over." Douggie goes
to the phone and calls the Host.
Oscar now has steam coming out of his nose.

After about ten minutes, the Casino Host approaches
Oscar and Mrs. Oscar.
I'm sure I'm paraphrasing the dialogue, but not being
a fly on the wall, it's the best I can do.

Host: Can I help you?
Oscar: Do I really have to go through this again?

More plaint and more litany.

Host: Do you have a Player's Card?

Oscar: No.

Host: Well, I can't check on how much gambling you've done unless you have a Player's Card.

Oscar: I haven't done any gambling. I didn't come here to gamble.

Host: Oh. Are you here for the tournament?

Oscar: No, I'm just here with my wife for some rest and relaxation.

Host: Then I don't think I can help you.

Oscar: But you're comping celebrities left and right! You comped Maury Povich for God's sake! Hell, I can buy and sell Maury Povich!

Host: (No longer having any reason to be nice, which is part of the job description)
Then you shouldn't have any trouble buying and selling this meal, should you.

Oscar: Why are you treating me like this?

Host: Sir, all of these celebrities, including Maury Povich, were invited here to play in the golf tournament. Comping their food is part of their deal.

It was beginning to sink in.
Oscar, sadly looking at the doggie bags, reached for his wallet, pulled out a credit card, and paid the check. And, according to Janine, left a very small tip.

So what have we learned? Once again, we've learned that Cheek is very unbecoming, and that an Academy Award will only get you so far.

*****

George Carlin, And The Prize He Should Have Won.

I watched George Carlin receive, posthumously, The Mark Twain Prize, on the PBS broadcast from the Kennedy Center. It was nice.
An earnest tribute from some of his peers, and many comedians whom he highly influenced.

But it made me sad.
Not only because it was posthumous.
I bet George would have loved to have been there, and revel in the fun tone of the evening.

The Mark Twain Prize always seemed to me to be the Booby Prize of entertainment awards.
Just a couple of steps above a Roast.

For many years, I've expressed my annoyance that the Kennedy Center Honors always went to members of down-the-middle mainstream and artsy-fartsy Show Business.
Too many ballerinas and violinists that nobody ever heard of that invariably lowered the ratings when their segments were on.
And WAY too many Country and Western singers.
Never to anybody who in the least bit smacked of controversy.
I would always use George Carlin as an example to anyone who asked.

To me, the Kennedy Center Honors Committee would finally make its bones when it honored George Carlin.
Now, it's too late.
They never honor anyone posthumously.

And what's the deal with them honoring foreigners?
I always thought that the Kennedy Honors had and should have a particularly American tone to them.

When Paul McCartney and Elton John were honored,
I was actually offended.
The way things have been lately, shouldn't we be
buying American?

It's not like they're running out of them.

In the mid 1980's, I was almost hired as David
Letterman's head writer. Their head writer was
leaving, and they were looking for a replacement.
My agent asked me if this would interest me.
I said "Hell, yeah!"
I was and am a huge Letterman fan.

As I only had a rep for writing sitcoms, I was asked to
submit some sample material.
A reasonable request.

That morning, I looked over the USA Today for topics
for monologue jokes.

I noticed that the Kennedy Center Honorees were
announced that day.

It was the year that Danny Kaye and Lena Horne were
honored.

I wrote the following joke for Dave (by that time, my
one-line snapper ability had increased significantly) :

"Did you hear that the Kennedy Center Honorees were
announced? They were Danny Kaye,
Lena Horne, _____, _____, and _____.
(I don't recall who the others were. I did at the time).
I don't know, five a year. That seems like a lot. You get
the feeling that they're going to run out of likely
candidates pretty soon.
I understand that for next year, they're going to take a
long, long look at Vic Tayback."

For those who don't remember, Vic Tayback played Mel of Mel's Diner on the TV series "Alice".

The joke went over well with Letterman.
I almost used Gavin McLeod.

My agent told me I was the only one they were considering from the outside.
It was either me, or they were promoting from within.
They promoted from within.
But I got to meet Dave and hear his flattering words about my material.
And I got to go home with one of those David Letterman yellow plastic collapsible drinking cups that he used to have on the show as MY Booby Prize.

But that was just a joke. They're not running out of good legitimate honorees.

I know that Carlin would have had fun at the Mark Twain Prize.
But he would have been so close to the real thing.

The event took place at the Kennedy Center, for chrissake!

Not even knowing him, I'd bet he would have wept at being a Kennedy Center Honoree.
But then, if you've been reading me often enough, you'd know that I'd bet on anything.

The outcome of his being a Kennedy Center honoree is that America would have grown up a little.

And he would have loved that.

He would have even shaken Bush's hand.
He would have been as cordial as Streisand was.

He would have even put on the tuxedo he wouldn't
allow himself to wear anymore in his Vegas act.
And wouldn't THAT have been something?!

Mort Sahl is still around.
He's in his eighties now.
Who knows how many more opportunities there are?

Maybe the Kennedy Center Committee can overlook
his even-now continuing swipes at the Warren
Commission, grow up, and honor him.

Even if you don't like the idea, you've got to admit it'd
be great drama.

*****

The Night Mort Sahl Broke My Heart.

I am, and have always been, a huge fan of Mort Sahl.

Mort Sahl was one of those trailblazers who changed the nature of Stand-Up Comedy.
He essentially bridged the gap between Alan King and Lenny Bruce.
Much more like the latter than the former.
Always topical.
Always literate.
Always playing to the top of our collective intelligence.
Always funny.
Very heady stuff.

Along the way, his career fell off the tracks when he got seriously involved with New Orleans D.A. Jim Garrison in his efforts to uncover a conspiracy in the JFK assassination.
He became a crusader in all his public appearances, much as Lenny Bruce had at the tail end of his career and life.
I completely sympathized with his point of view about the Kennedy assassination.
I still do.

He eventually got his bearings, and returned to the comedy he did best, which was political commentary.

With the change from the Alan Kings and all the "Jackie's" and "Joeys" and "Hennys" and "Sheckys" of comedy to the Mort Sahls and Lenny Bruces and George Carlins and Richard Pryors was one key element:
The former group was doing routines.
The latter group was telling us the truth.

Truth was a vital element in their presentation.

They were all essentially preaching the gospel as they saw it.
Or at least as the audience perceived it.
And it was a major part of their appeal.

There was an implied contract with the audience that these latter day comedians thoroughly believed what they were saying.
And the audience loved them for it.

Carlin risked his career for it.
Lenny Bruce gave up his life for it.

Unfortunately, Mort Sahl, who risked his career for other, perhaps more important reasons,
risked nothing for his comedy, including the truth.

Now, this might seem like a small thing to you as I describe it, but when I experienced it, it seemed like an absolute breach of faith.

I was in Las Vegas. I think it was in the late 70's.

Mort Sahl was playing at the Lounge of the Hilton Hotel.
I had never seen him work live, and I was staying at the Hilton.

I couldn't pass up the opportunity.
He did a great set. The kind he used to do in his prime before the Kennedy mishegoss.
It was wonderful.
So wonderful that I went back the next night to catch him again.

That's when it happened.
It was mostly the same material. I guess he didn't expect there to be much repeat business.

He launched into a story that he had told the night before about appearing on the Merv Griffin Show.

I forget the point of the story, but as he told it, he was sitting next to Donna Reed on Merv's couch, holding her up to be a bastion of wholesomeness, and mildly putting her down for it.

That's how he told it the first night.
The second night, he changed Donna Reed to Debbie Reynolds.

I don't think it was a lapse of memory.
I think he thought, "I think I can get a bigger laugh with Debbie Reynolds."

At that moment, Mort Sahl proved to me that he was full of shit.
And it broke my heart.

Jack Paar, when occasionally telling some outlandish story on his show and sensing that the audience was skeptical, would stop and say "Look, if we don't have trust, we have nothing".
I've subsequently learned from people who wrote for Paar that he only rarely flirted with the truth.

Mort Sahl doesn't have the right to be full of shit.
Alan King did.
Mort Sahl doesn't.

That night in Vegas was like seeing the King without his clothes on.
But as ugly as he was naked, he's still a King.
Alan King wasn't.
Mort Sahl is.

*****

Hire The Handicapped.

This is going to be yet another version of "Agents are scum."

After all this time, and so many examples, you wouldn't necessarily think that there could be yet another version of "Agents are scum."

But they constantly surprise you with the depths they are capable of reaching.

They did, a couple of months ago, with me.

In putting together my movie, I wanted to check on the availability of an actress I had worked with many times.

A wonderful actress.
She's done a lot of TV, and you may or may not recognize her name, depending on how closely you follow credits.
I'm not going to make any effort to help you on that score.

I knew that she has had some minor health problems lately.
The kind that have a "major health problem" label attached to them.
She has been fairly open about these problems.

I was advised about who her agent was, and I made the call.
Some young voice on the other end of the phone said she'd never heard of her.
I said "You represent her."
She said "I know who we represent, and we don't represent her".
I said "I have very reliable information that indicates that you do."

She said "You're starting to waste my time."
I said "Are you sure we're talking about the same person?"

Then I started rattling off her TV credits.
Then I mentioned the "disease" she has.

The voice on the other end of the phone then said "Ohhhh! You want the Handicapped Department! Why didn't you say so?"

Why didn't I say so.
Why on earth would I think to say so?!

Why on earth would I think that a talent agency would have a "Handicapped" department for some of their clients?
Isn't this some sort of illegal discrimination?

And why on earth wouldn't the rest of the agency be apprised of the talent pool that comprised the "Handicapped Department"?

Could it possibly be because they didn't give a crap?!

Because how much income could their "Handicapped Department" provide for them anyway?

They connected me to the Handicapped Department.
The Handicapped Department had indeed heard of the actress I was inquiring about.
I spoke to someone, left my phone number and asked for the actress in question to give me a call.
They took down the information, and said "We can't promise anything."
Would it matter if they did?
What good have their promises ever been?

The next day, the actress in question called me.
I mentioned my interest in possibly having her be in my movie.

She seemed enthused.

Then I said something that was perhaps none of my business, but I was just trying to be helpful.
I asked if she knew that she was only listed by her agency as being in the Handicapped Department.

She didn't even know what that was.
They hadn't even asked or told her about it.

I told her how difficult it was to even confirm that she was their client, until by pure luck, it was established that she was in the Handicapped Department.

This was certainly disheartening for her.
I asked her what she was going to do about it.

She said "Probably nothing. It wouldn't be easy for me to get another agent, the way things are. I don't really want to piss them off."
I volunteered that it's virtually like she doesn't have an agent now.

Eventually, I found out that she got brave enough to make enough of a stink to get herself out of the Handicapped Department.

I wonder if anyone who's considered to be in the Handicapped Department was apprised of their status.
Or that there even is a Handicapped Department.

I used to operate under the delusion that these people were supposed to operate in your best interests.

I've known better for quite a while now.

This is one of the major reasons I live in Michigan. Although, as the movie industry is moving in a big way to Michigan, I'm pretty sure the scum will follow.
*****

Does Anybody Here Speak English?

I had one of my Wednesday jaunts into Manhattan yesterday to see a couple of shows.
I just want to relate to you the absolute highlight of my day.
Because it isn't every day that I get to make a public spectacle of myself.
That's primarily because I don't get out in public all that often.

It was about 1:15 pm, and I had some time to kill before the 2 o'clock matinee.
So I went to the eighth floor lounge at the Marriott Marquis in Times Square to hang out for about twenty minutes.
There weren't many seats available, so it was pretty much either stand and loiter, or sit next to two men seated at a table, conversing.
One of them was conversing very loudly. The other barely opened his mouth.

It became apparent very quickly that the man doing all the talking was interviewing the other man for a job.
It was a job as a salesman/telemarketer for what the talkative one said was the Number One Insect Repellant Manufacturer in the Country.
I know this because he referred to it that way about five times.
He said EVERYTHING he said about five times.

I felt really badly for this well-dressed poor sap who was being interviewed.
This poor Hispanic well-dressed sap.
I assume he was Hispanic because he looked it, and the other guy kept calling him Jose.

I thought what I usually thought: That without the breaks I've gotten, I could have been a Jewish version of this poor well-dressed sap. There but for the Grace of God.......

The interviewer was all well-dressed sleaze.
Picture Alec Baldwin in "GlenGarry GlenRoss".
Only without the charm.

You just knew that EVERYTHING the man was saying was complete bullshit.
"We won't be able to let you know for at least a couple of weeks whether we'll be hiring you because we have many, many applicants....".
Yeah.
Applicants are just breaking down this guy's door for a straight commission job as an Insect Repellant Salesman/Telemarketer.
He probably didn't even have a door to break down.
Or why would he be conducting this interview, embarrassing this poor sap, in public, at the top of his voice, not buying him anything to eat, at lunchtime?
He called himself the Vice-President.
The Vice-President of the Number One Insect Repellant Manufacturing Company is interviewing some poor sap as a Salesman/Telemarketer?
In public?
Gee, you'd think he'd at least have an office or something.

This was the sentence that led to my making a public spectacle of myself:
"You know, this company has a lot of turnaround. Employees come and go."

"Turnaround"?

I believe the word anyone with a reasonable command of the language would use is "Turnover".

As a writer, I consider myself to be a guardian of the language.
So the second time he said this sentence, the hairs on the back of my neck began rising.

On the third and fourth pass, my anger was steadily mounting.

On the fifth, I found myself, virtually unconsciously, blurting out "TURNOVER!!!!" in his direction.
He looked at me huffily and said, huffily, "Excuse me?!!"

"TURNOVER!! TURNOVER!! Not 'turnaround'!! TURNOVER!!

I rose, leaned over him, stared at him, and said, at full volume, just like Burt Lancaster in "The Rainmaker" said about water, "English!! I recommend it!!"

I turned on a dime, not waiting for a response, or seeing one, strutted out of there, and headed for the theatre.

Great way to start the day, hah?

*****

Ricky Nelson Was Wrong.

In the early 70's, Ricky Nelson participated in an early
Rock' n Roll revival concert at Madison Square
Garden, along with quite a few other notables from
that era.
After singing a few of his old hits, he then sang
something new that he had written.
Something in another style, and something the
audience had never heard of, and didn't want to hear
of.
He then was booed off the stage.

As a result of this bitter experience, he wrote a bitter
Hit Song called "Garden Party".

Here are many of the lyrics to "Garden Party":

"I went to a garden party
To reminisce with my old friends
A chance to share old memories
And play our songs again

When I got to the garden party
They all knew my name
No one recognized me
I didn't look the same

But it's all right now
I learned my lesson well
You see, ya can't please everyone
So ya got to please yourself

People came from miles around
Everyone was there
Yoko brought her walrus
There was magic in the air

Played them all the old songs
Thought that's why they came
No one heard the music
We didn't look the same

I said hello to 'Mary Lou
She belongs to me
When I sang a song about a honky-tonk
It was time to leave

Someone opened up a closet door
And out stepped Johnny B Goode
Playing guitar
Like a-ringin' a bell
And lookin' like he should

If you gotta play at garden parties
I wish you a lotta luck
But if memories were all I sang
I rather drive a truck

But it's all right now
I learned my lesson well
You see, ya can't please everyone
So ya got to please yourself......."

"If memories were all I sang, I'd rather drive a truck".

This past Saturday Night, I got to see a lot of people who would rather sing just memories than drive a truck.
As would most of us.

I went to a Doo-Wop Concert in Detroit, after being invited by my nephew and niece, both in their mid-twenties.

It was held in an outdoor amphitheatre that held about 2,000 people, and was a little more than half-filled.

I understand that last year, when they held it, it was completely filled.
That it wasn't this year was a little discouraging.
No matter.
It was fabulous.
The audience was mostly my age, but, gratifyingly, there were quite a few people my niece and nephew's age.

Most of the groups were just vaguely known to me by name, and there were certainly some replacements, but many of the lead singers were the originals, or at least in on the ground floor of these groups.
And I certainly knew their big hits, which is what they all sang.
Among others:

The Zodiacs---"Stay", before the Four Seasons did it, and "Little Darlin", before The Diamonds did it.

Cleve Duncan and the Penguins---"Earth Angel"

The Vogues--"Turn Around, Look At Me", "My Special Angel"

The Clovers--"Devil Or Angel", "Love Potion Number Nine"

And they brought out Jimmy Clanton, not exactly Doo-Wop, but he had a few hits----
"Go Jimmy, Go", "Venus In Blue Jeans", "Just a Dream".
And he was still adorable, with a huge shock of white hair.

This thing was organized really well.
People were clapping along and dancing in the aisles from the beginning, including me.
And they built it great to set up the Headliners: The Drifters.

Just their entrance caused pandemonium.
The lead singer was in great voice.
They opened with "This Magic Moment".

The audience was theirs.

Then "Save The Last Dance For Me".

Putty. We were putty.

"On Broadway".

Jelly. We were jelly.

"Up On The Roof"

Liquid.

And they finished with the combination one-two
punch of "There Goes My Baby", and, of course,
closing with "Under The Boardwalk".

The 1200 or so people in the audience were in tears.

They brought everyone back at the end and they all
sang "Good Night Sweetheart, Well It's Time To Go".

We were all wiped out.

You have to please everyone.
You can't just please yourself.

What I was witnessing and experiencing were
everyone on stage, and many in the audience, re-living
the happiest moments of their lives.

Maybe if he had lived, Ricky would have realized that
you don't get this from driving a truck.

*****

That's All, Rose.

If you remember Carl Ballantine, who died not too long ago, you probably best remember him as one of the crew of the 60's sitcom "McHale's Navy".

This is unfortunate.
It was easily the weakest of his work.

It was easily the weakest work of any actor connected with any other show.

"McHale's Navy" was what is known in the trade, or at least in my house, as a Bad Sitcom.

They essentially tried to do "Sergeant Bilko", wet.

At least they were aspiring to greatness.
But they did some bad hiring.

The Executive Producer of "Bilko" was someone named Edward J. Montaigne.
If they had been able to read through the cracks of the credits, the powers that be would have realized that Montaigne was simply the Line Producer. The Nuts and Bolts guy.

The creative muscle of "Bilko" was the genius Nat Hiken.
He was nowhere to be found.
They hired Edward J. Montaigne to recapture the "Bilko" magic.
And Montaigne went out and hired a lot of bad writers.
And turned out a very embarrassing, idiotic, repetitious, silly show.
It was inherently stupid. the one thing I can't abide.

What an incredibly wasteful use of wonderful actors.
At least Montaigne cast well.

He even cast Billy Sands, who was Private Papparelli on "Bilko", where he was always funny, and made him one of the crew for McHale, where he was never funny.

He had the great Tim Conway, and had him be relentlessly silly.
He had Ernest Borgnine, who subsequently demonstrated a great flair for comedy, but not on that show.
It was all because of what Garry Marshall called RR. Rotten Writing.

And it had Carl Ballantine, who actually transcended the RR, and WAS funny.

Those of you who are a little older might remember The Amazing Ballantine:
Carl as the world's worst magician.
He must have done it at least 20 times on the Ed Sullivan Show.
You can find it on YouTube.
It was my introduction to him, and I laugh just thinking about it.
It was the domestic forerunner to Dom DeLuise's "Dominick The Great", and quite similar to it.
Whether Dom committed theft or homage, I'm glad he did it.

To me, the height of Carl Ballantine's impact on comedy was several guest appearances on "Car 54, Where Are You?", which WAS run by the great Nat Hiken.

"Car 54" starred Joe E. Ross (from "Bilko"), who played Gunther Toody, a New York patrol car cop, and Fred Gwynne, who played Francis Muldoon, his partner. Gwynne also cut his teeth on a couple of episodes of "Bilko".

"Car 54" was ALWAYS hilarious.

In a handful of episodes, Gunther's wife Lucille
(played by the same actress who played Joe E. Ross's
wife on "Bilko", Hiken kept drawing from the same
well.) invited her sister Rose and Rose's husband Al
over for dinner.
Lucille's attitude towards Gunther was contempt, and
"Why can't you be more like Al?"
Al was played by Carl Ballantine.

Rose and Al would come over. Al would immediately
plop down on the couch light up a cigar, and bury his
head in a newspaper, ignoring everyone else.
Rose would then begin prattling on about how
wonderful Al was in general----
"Oh, I'm so lucky. Nobody is as lucky as I am. Al is just
the sweetest, most loving, most giving husband a girl
could wish for.
Last week, it was my birthday, and Al took me to a
Chinese restaurant. An actual Chinese restaurant.
With fortune cookies and everything......"
And from behind the newspaper, you'd hear
Carl Ballantine's voice, saying "That's all, Rose."

And Rose would immediately clam up.
In mid-sentence.

The evening would go along, and Rose would again
start prattling about how wonderful Al was,
and after the duly alotted time, Al would again cut her
off with "That's all, Rose", and she'd immediately shut
up.

It usually happened 3 or 4 times each episode, and
occurred in each episode they appeared in.

They just don't write 'em like that anymore.
The furthest thing from RR that one could imagine.

About six years later, I was in college, directing one of the skits for the frat and sorority competitions we were involved in. I'd described them previously.

We were paired with a very whiny girls group. Nobody was happy with what we were doing, and the girls were very vocal about it.
This one girl was particularly vocal about it.
This girl was considered a barometer of sorts.
She was right on the borderline of good-looking and not good-looking.
If you were better looking than she, you were good-looking.
If you were any worse looking than she, you were bad-looking.
It was that simple.
Anyway, she kept yammering on.
If she was any worse looking, I probably would have put an end to it sooner.
But like I said, she was right on the borderline.
Finally I couldn't take anymore.
Oh, and her name was Rose.
And I said "That's all, Rose".

The guys, who all knew the reference, were doubled up in laughter, and toppling all over each other, giggling uncontrollably.

And, of course, Rose didn't get it.
"What's so funny?" "Why is everybody laughing at me?", she said in her whiny, marginally attractive voice.
I tried to explain, but some things just can't help but be lost in the translation.

R.I.P., Carl.

*****

The Funny Man We Lost This Week.

As far as I'm concerned, Lionel Stander was one of the Top Ten funniest actors I've ever seen.

I began casting for a pilot in 1976 for a sitcom which became a series called "Busting Loose".
It was basically an attempt by CBS to do its version of the hit movie "Next Stop, Greenwich Village".
It ended up being a slightly Jewish contemporary version of "Happy Days".
It was pretty funny.
And only slightly Jewish because networks have been traditionally gun-shy about doing anything overtly Jewish once people in Wyoming got TV sets.
But early on in the process, it started out being much more Jewish than it ended up.
And there was a need for a Jewish father for his son, the lead, who turned out to be Adam Arkin.

I had a major Jones going to cast Lionel Stander.
I thought he'd be great.
I had lunch with him and his very young wife, and tried to talk him into it.
He was reluctant.
My heart was broken when he turned me down.

Lionel Stander died 15 years ago, so this isn't about him.

We held regular auditions to fill Lionel's shoes.
We saw a lot of bad old Jewish actors.

Then, a wonderful actor named Jack Kruschen came into the room and was quite delightful.
Personally and acting-wise.
You might remember him as the doctor in the movie "The Apartment".

He was nominated for an Oscar for that.
This isn't about him either.
Jack died years ago.

But we cast him, and he was just dandy.
That was the problem.
He was JUST dandy.
No more than JUST.

And about ten minutes after we signed him, I thought
of who I really wanted.
Even more than Lionel Stander.

What I thought I'd get with Lionel Stander was
someone who'd lift up the entire stage when he'd
enter a scene.
Lionel would have done that.
But not nearly as well as Lou Jacobi would.

That's who died this week. The last week in October
of 2009.
One of the five funniest actors I've ever seen.
And that's who I should have thought of originally.
If we'd had him, maybe the show would have stayed
more Jewish.
And who knows, maybe even be successful.

Jack Kruschen never lifted up the stage when he
entered.
He was more than competent, but couldn't bring
enough to the part so that CBS didn't want to cut
down on his screen time.
That's what ended up happening.
Lou Jacobi wouldn't have let that happen.
Through sheer force of will, presence, ability, and the
funniness of his bones.

If this all sounds familiar, it's basically the same situation I ran into when we cast Phil Foster in "Laverne and Shirley", and then I realized I wanted Frankie Laine.

You'd think you'd learn from your mistakes.
No.

I've seen four different versions of "The Sunshine Boys", not counting the atrocity of a TV movie that Woody Allen and Peter Falk did, when Neil Simon decided to fix what wasn't broke.
I'm talking about three on Broadway, and the original movie.
The three on Broadway who played Al Lewis were Sam Levene (opposite Jack Albertson),
Lou Jacobi (opposite Jack Gilford), and Tony Randall (opposite Jack Klugman).
And, of course, in the movie it was George Burns (opposite Walter Matthau).
None of these men could be described as slouches.
Each one a shtarker in his own right.

None of the others could touch Lou Jacobi.
He made lines funny that nobody else made funny.
His timing was unmatched.
He just oozed funny.

His acting style was that of "pronouncement".
He pronounced his lines, rather than saying them.
But in a quite believable manner.
There's a five minute clip of him on YouTube as a judge, doing what is essentially a monologue, even though there are other people in the courtroom, in the movie "Little Murders".
Treat yourself to it.

When I've directed, I've often told actors that I want
certain lines "pronounced".
Actually, that was code for "Do it like Lou Jacobi".

For those of you who lived in New York in the 60's,
you might remember that he did a commercial for
Levy's Real Jewish Rye Bread.
He played a grocer, and did this monologue into the
telephone:

"Yes Mrs. Brown. Levy's Real Jewish Rye Bread. I'll
have it for you tomorrow......(we hear the buzzing of
Mrs. Brown's complaining coming out of the
phone.)....Tomorrow, I'll have it for you.
(More phone complaining)......tomorrow.
Tomorrow.....to-morr-row."

Doesn't sound like much on paper.
In his hands, it was a three act play, written by
everyone in Sid Caesar's writers room.

He lived to be 95.

Proof that there is a God.

*****

The Other Funny Man We Lost This Week. (Same Week)

Like millions and millions of others, I loved Soupy Sales.

Between my wife and me, we have virtually seen Soupy's entire career, even though most of it was spent in local television.

Our perspectives are a little different.

My wife is about eight years younger than I am, and grew up in Detroit, which is where Soupy broke in "Lunch with Soupy Sales". It was on there Monday through Saturday at noon.

This was in 1961, when my wife was six.

In New York, where I grew up, it only aired on Saturdays.

I didn't even know it was on all week in Detroit until she told me.

So she got to see a lot of the early stuff as a little kid, and I didn't.

What I saw, I loved.

The only problem I had was his choice of food for his lunch.

He'd usually have a bologna sandwich, or a hot dog, with a glass of milk.

Growing up in a semi-kosher home, this seemed rather repulsive.

Then, for dessert, he always had Jello.

One of his sponsors.

He would tap at the Jello, which came out of a Jello mold. It would always wiggle, and you'd hear the "Boi-oi-oi-oi-oing" sound effect.

Then, a few years later, Soupy moved his act to New York, was on at 3:30 in the afternoon, and, being too

late for lunch, no longer had it and no longer repulsed
me.
This was definitely an upgrade.
Although I did miss the Jello tapping.

I got to see him every weekday after school.
But my wife completely lost touch with Soupy.
He wasn't on there anymore.

What she had lost, I had gained.

I got to witness whatever "evolving" went on.
There wasn't much, but there was some.
He started doing "The Mouse", and got a hit record
out of it.

He also started doing the "Philo Kvetch" sketch, which
was a low point.

In any case, Soupy was a genuine trailblazer.
He was a high-wire act, working with no writers, no
budget, working almost totally off the cuff.
Playing to the crew, the same thing as playing to the
band, even though he didn't have one, using puppets
extensively, and being relentlessly funny.

High wire act? No writers? No budget? Off the cuff?
Playing to the band even though he didn't have one?
Relentlessly funny? Rotten sketches? Using puppets
extensively?......Remind you of anyone?

Craig Ferguson, wittingly or not, has taken up the
mantle.
Give him a few pies, have people come to the door
where you only see their hands,
and you've got Soupy. With a Scottish accent.

Soupy also introduced me to some of the great
comedy albums of the time when he'd check the
"Weather Report" on the radio.

I'd hear Stan Freberg, and people like Eddie
Lawrence, "The Old Philosopher", for the first time.
Soupy really expanded my horizons.
He made life better for all of us.
Seeing him, and just thinking about him.

Mark Goodson, the prolific game show producer, was
asked who his favorite panelist was.
Without batting an eyelash, he said Soupy Sales.
"He brought more entertainment value than anyone
else I ever had".

I remember when Soupy was a regular panelist on the
syndicated version of "What's My Line?", where they
didn't wear tuxedos and evening gowns.
They did a running segment where they would bring
four people out of the audience, and the panelists
would have to match the people with their
occupations by holding big cards in front of them,
indicating their occupations.
Most of the panelists got it wrong , including Soupy.
But when Soupy got it wrong, he would invariably
turn to the camera, in a shot that contained him and
the contestants, and thrusted his fists downward in a
gesture that indicated "Drat!"
He would do this EVERY TIME.
I don't know if anyone else noticed, but it slayed me
every time.

Since the 1970's, I have performed an annual ritual
involving my sister, Leslie.

At some point in the 70's, our grandmother passed
away.
Prior to this occurrence, on our respective birthdays,
our grandmother would call us on the phone and sing
"Happy Birthday To You".
With her heavy Yiddish accent.
She used to write letters to people in English, with a
heavy Yiddish accent in the writing.

She had, long prior to this, Yiddishized our names.
I was Macchinyu.
To paraphrase Johnny Cash, life ain't easy for a boy
named Macchinyu.

My sister was Leslincocinunchicl.
That ain't any easier.

So on my sister's birthday, it was always
"Heppy Boiseday tooh yooh,
Heppy Boiseday tooh yooh,
Heppy Boiseday Leslincocinunchicl,
Heppy Boiseday tooh yooh."

Then she died, and it was over.

But something came over me to not let this tradition
die with her.

So from then on, every year, I would call my sister on
her birthday, doing a dead on imitation of my
grandmother singing her rendition of "Heppy
Boiseday".
It was always well received.

After a few years of this, in order to avoid repetition,
I'd start doing riffs off of the general concept.
I'd do a jazz rendition. A calypso version, a semi-
operatic version----you get the idea.

Then, I stumbled across the notion of mimicking
celebrities mimicking my grandmother singing
"Heppy Boiseday" to my sister.
My first endeavor was as Marilyn Monroe, singing a
very breathy "Heppy Boiseday", much as she sang to
Kennedy at his very public birthday party.

But heavily Yiddishified.
It went over very big.

I have a very good ear for mimickry, so every year, it was another celebrity imitating my grandmother singing "Heppy Boiseday".
I started out with the old standards, Cagney, Bogart, Edward G. Robinson, Cary Grant.

Then it got a little more exotic. The highlights of my work included Neil Diamond, Willie Nelson and Julio Iglesias in tandem---"For All The Boisedays You've Had Before...."

Rodney Dangerfield was a big hit.

Then, a couple of years ago, I decided to do Soupy Sales, White Fang, and Black Tooth.

Some of these involve more structure than others.
I decided to create a scenario where Soupy was going to sing the song, but was interrupted by White Fang and Black Tooth, who both complained that they had more of a right to sing the song because they were far better Jews than Soupy was.
White Fang would ask, in his gibberished way, how often Soupy went to shul.
Soupy was forced to admit that he really only went on the High Holidays.
White Fang replied "Wehh ooo wehhh wehhh oo wehh ehh"
Soupy would answer "Really? Every shabbos?"
Turns out White Fang and Black Tooth were Orthodox.
This was too much for Soupy to offer a cogent argument against.
So he relented, and allowed White Fang and Black Tooth to sing "Heppy Boiseday" to my sister, in their relative incoherency.

I performed this little playlet in that year's phone call.
My sister had it on the speaker phone, and her husband heard it as well.

They were both blown away, and to this day, it has
been a hard act to follow.

Her husband had the most interesting reaction.
It was, essentially that anyone could do White Fang
and Black Tooth like that, but he had never heard
anyone nail Soupy like I did.

What he was not privy to was that since I first met my
wife about twenty years ago, and realized our mutual
love for each other and Soupy, literally not a day has
gone by where one or both of us has not lapsed into a
vocal impression of Soupy.
So I had plenty of practice nailing Soupy.

When Soupy would say "Kids, now it's time to check
out the Words of Wisdom, cause it's very impot'nt...."
that would translate in our house into "And now it's
time to take out the garbage, cause it's very
impotn't...."
Or I'd ask my wife if she'd make me breakfast.
She'd say okay, and I'd say "and you do dat, I love you
give big kiss".

The man was not without influence.

I'll bet Soupy had a wonderful life. I'm sure there
some who experienced it more extensively because
they had more national exposure throughout their
careers, but there were only a handful of people who
made such a positive impact on their audience, adults
and kids, that every time they walked down the street,
people whom they didn't know were glad to see them,
and told them regularly.
Soupy was certainly one of the people who had this
particular perk.   This is my definition of a great life.

*****

The Doctor And The Rounds Girl.

It was the late 70's. I was the show runner of one of my One-Season Wonders.
I'm not sure I even remember which one.

I was experiencing chest and stomach pains.
All around me were cajoling me to make a doctor's appointment.
Being easily cajoled, as much as I generally despised doctors and still do, I made one.

So I show up, and they put me through a battery of tests.
They give me e.k.g.'s, have me drink barium in order to X-Ray me for a possible ulcer, and
begin the X-Ray process.

So there I am, in the X-Ray room, wearing a hospital gown, with my ass sticking out, standing up next to the machine, and getting X-Rayed.

The middle-aged nurse enters the room, pushing in a long table, with a big sheet covering its contents.
Another nurse, a young very pretty one, is with her.

The middle-aged nurse says to me, alluding to the other nurse, "This is my sister Sandi.
She's not really a nurse".
I say "Really? She's dressed like a nurse."
"I'm not really a nurse," pipes up Sandi.
"I'm an actress."
"Really?" I inquire.
"Well, I'd like to be", she replies.

Now, let's step back and momentarily examine the dynamics of the situation.

I was trapped. Ambushed.

My only option was to be polite.

"Well, have you had any experience?", I asked.

"Oh, I've been on television many times ".

"Really? (With my ass hanging out) Anything I might have seen?"

"Do you ever watch ABC's Wide World of Sports?"
"Sure."
"CBS Sports Spectacular?"
"Yes"
"NBC Sportsworld?"
"Often. You must be an athlete".
"No. I'm the Rounds Girl. At Caesar's Palace"

I'm now starting to feel like George Burns playing straight for Gracie Allen.
The difference being that my ass was hanging out.

"The Rounds Girl?

"Yeah. At the fights. Between rounds, I walk around the ring holding up this big card saying what round it is."
"Oh."
"You know. Like Round 2, or Round 3......."
"Or Round 4 or Round 5?" I add.
"Exactly".

She then proceeds to remove the sheet from the long table, revealing a television set, hooked up to a VCR.
She plugs them in.
She turns on the VCR, showing me her highlight reel as the Caesar's Palace Rounds Girl.

She looks at me, with all the soulfulness her eyes could muster, and said "I'd do anything to get a part on one of your shows. And I mean ANYTHING.

I must admit I was wavering. I was after all, human. But nothing came of it.

I received what seemed to be a rather urgent call from the doctor's office the next week to set up an immediate appointment. They had the results of my tests.
This scared the crap out of me. What did they find?
I asked "Can't you tell me over the phone?
"No, the doctor must see you personally".

I show up two days later, the earliest he could squeeze me in.
With my heart in my mouth, he tells me that all the tests showed that I was fine.
Just a little gas.
After experiencing major relief, I got very angry, and released this anger on the doctor.
"You mean you scared the shit out of me by insisting to see me in person to tell me this?
Just to collect a fee for an office visit?"
Doctors don't like to be talked to like this, but he didn't really have a good response.
I left his office, calling him a "Cocksucker", or some such epithet.
This is what the Health Care Industry in this country has deteriorated FROM.

Several weeks later, I was sitting at home watching a fight on ABC's Wide World of Sports, and it was between Rounds 7 and 8, and, by God, there was Sandi, walking around the ring carrying the big card that said "Round 8".

At least some people are on the up and up.
*****

Jean Simmons Movie Star.

In the early 1960's, they used to run a public service commercial in New York.
It was usually on late at night.
There was this little boy, and an even littler girl sitting in front of a stoop, bouncing a ball beteen them. And the dialogue between them would go as follows:

Girl: Mayor Wagner does?

Boy: Mayor Wagner does.

Girl: Jackie Robinson does?

Boy: Jackie Robinson does.

Girl: Even Sam Lemonson?

Boy: (Haughtily and derisively) You mean Sam Levenson!

Girl: Sam Levenson REALLY does?

Boy Sam Levenson really does
.
Girl: Dina Merrill Movie Star does?

Boy: Uh huh.

It turns out that what they all do is throw their litter into litter baskets on the streets of New York, rather than toss it willy-nilly on to the ground.
It was their anti-littering campaign.
It ends with the announcer saying "9 out of 10 New Yorkers do. How about you?"

Now, this would have gone totally unremembered by me, except for that little girl saying
"Dina Merrill Movie Star does?"
Some ad copywriter actually WROTE that.

This was the best way they could figure for them to cover the fact that a little girl could have possibly heard of Dina Merrill, and provide a sop to Dina Merrill to get her to participate in this ad.

Dina Merrill, to my knowledge, never was a movie star.

She appeared in movies, but was never what you might call a star.
It ends with all named in a still picture tossing litter into a basket, One of them being Dina (Is there anyone feena?)
.
But they had that little girl say "Dina Merrill Movie Star does?"
This is the kind of thing that sticks with you.
It deserves its own wing in the Cheeziness Hall of Fame.

From shortly thereafter to the present, every movie star you can think of has been referred to as "_____
_____ Movie Star" by select cronies of mine, and of course, myself.

The first time it was actually said, though not within earshot, in the presence of an actual movie star, was the first day of my professional writing career.

Jean Simmons was in the rehearsal hall where "The Odd Couple" was experiencing the first reading of the script she was to guest star in.
Our immediate reaction: "It's Jean Simmons Movie Star".

Except she really was one.

Jean Simmons was really quite something.
Remember her in "Spartacus", with Kirk Douglas
Movie Star?
She just radiated on the screen.
Or "Elmer Gantry", where she was just marvelous
opposite Burt Lancaster Movie Star?
And she was just delightful to be around.

When everyone broke for lunch that first day, some of
us, including me and Jean Simmons Movie Star went
to the Paramount commissary, then widely known for
having the worst food on earth.

The restaurants that were in the immediate
neighborhood were only marginally better.

One of them provided an entrance through the
kitchen, where stacks of canned vegetables were on
display. It was as if they were practically advertising
"We just don't give a shit."

One time, at one of the other movie studios, a meeting
broke up, it was dinnertime, and one of the
participants actually suggested that we all get in our
cars and DRIVE to this restaurant for dinner.
To me, this was unfathomable, and I lost what little
respect I had for this individual.

So with only an hour for lunch that day, it made just
about as much sense to eat at the godawful
commissary.
Jean Simmons Movie Star was seated at a table by
herself when I entered.
I didn't know if this was by choice, and I summoned
up the nerve to ask her if she'd like company.

I knew she wouldn't like the food. I was offering

myself up as a possible consolation prize.
She seemed delighted that anyone took the trouble to
pay any attention to her.

I got my dreadful meal, returned to her table and sat
down and shot the shit with Jean Simmons Movie
Star for an hour.
It was so delightful that we barely noticed that we
were both probably being slowly poisoned.
That Friday night, she was absolutely charming acting
primarily opposite Jack Klugman TV Star.

Then, two years later, the ultimate irony.
You know who did a guest shot on "The Odd Couple"
as Oscar's love interest?
You got it in one guess.
Dina Merrill Movie Star.

I didn't bring it up. I just spent the entire week stifling
a giggle and keeping my trap shut.

*****

Coming Soon:

"Mark Rothman's Essays. Volume 2.

"Mark Rothman's Report Cards: A collection of film and stage reviews in a unique style."

For further information, e-mail Mark at macchus999@aol.com

*****